PRAISE FOR THE PO
NO

"Sue has done a brilliant job of breaking down the mechanics of what it takes to be successful in any area of your life so it can be easily duplicated by anyone! Her ability to explain complex subjects like Quantum Physics, Brain Science and Epigenetics in a way that people of all ages can comprehend is fantastic! I highly recommend this book to anyone who wants to finally break free from the shackles of their old life and step into a beautiful, meaningful and fulfilling next chapter of their life."

NATALIE LEDWELL

Best Selling Author and Founder of Mind Movies

"Sue Stone's brilliant new book, "The Power Within You Now", is a life changer. She explains simply and clearly how you can create love, prosperity, success, peace or whatever you want in your life and includes the scientific research that demonstrates how the techniques work. Sue shares her own experiences and how she has learnt to fine-tune different exercises to make them more effective. By following them she has created a rich and abundant life for herself and her family. There is a resonance of truth about this book and if you follow the guidelines you too can make your dreams come true."

DIANA COOPER

World Spiritual Teacher & Author

"The Power Within You Now" provides an excellent and clear overview on how to build the life you desire in a way that will enrich your mind, body and soul. On top of Sue's relatable story and her ability to distil life-changing advice into simple directives, Sue takes great care to explain HOW it all works on a scientific level in a way you can easily understand and implement into your daily life."

MATTHEW TOMAN & DANIEL HOLMES

Co-creators of "The Evolution of Success"

"Sue Stone's latest book is a brilliant life guide for everyone from millennials to baby boomers. It is full of tips and insights gained from Sue's own experiences and informed scientific based research to help you raise your spirits, manifest your needs and dreams and reclaim your personal power. A great and easy read that should be available in every school to teach our children how to develop and consciously manage and create positive feelings, beliefs and mindsets."

ANNE JONES

International Speaker, Author and Healer

THE POWER WITHIN YOU NOW!

Rocket fuel for your mind, body & soul

BY SUE STONE

First published in June 2019

A catalogue record for this book is available from the British Library.

Paperback ISBN: 9780955833014

About the Author

Sue Stone of the Sue Stone Foundation is a happiness and empowerment leader and business mentor. She is an international motivational and inspirational speaker and is available for talks, seminars and workshops worldwide.

She is regularly on TV and radio, including Channel 4s Secret Millionaire and How'd You Get So Rich.

In 2011 Sue set up the Sue Stone Foundation to truly make a difference across the world. She has a growing global team of Accredited Coaches within the SSF, who give one to one and group workshop sessions and talks. These encompass an expansive range of personal obstacles and challenges that are faced by individuals from all walks of life.

For contact details, other products available or to book Sue please visit www.suestone.com.

To join Sue's team in the Sue Stone Foundation or to find an accredited coach to help you please visit www.suestonefoundation.com.

CONTENTS

INTRODUCTION

My intention with this book is to share what has profoundly and positively changed *my* life and the lives of so many others.

My interest is to prove to people that they have within their reach all the tools necessary to make significant changes in their bodies and in their lives.

I have endeavoured to take complex scientific information and to simplify it in a way that is translatable and useable in our daily lives. The more people understand how and why this 'stuff' works, what they are doing and why they are doing it, the 'how' gets easier.

I haven't been on any personal development courses and I don't possess a PhD in psychology or a Masters degree in biology, physics or chemistry. What I do possess is 2 decades of self-study and applying what I discovered into my life.

When you understand that you are not bound by the chains of your past, all things truly become possible.

Throughout the book I have deliberately used repetition to reinforce some points, as reiterating and re-affirming makes it much more likely that the ideas and concepts will stick.

I am passionate about bridging the gap between science, spirituality and the material worlds. You may find that certain chapters resonate more than others at this moment in time and that is perfectly fine.

I am purely sharing what has helped me totally transform my life at every level and I hope it will provide the rocket fuel to ignite you so you too can create a life you love and beyond!

Sue Stone

CONNECT WITH ME:

I love being in touch with my readers

Facebook.com/SueStoneOfficial
Instagram.com/suestoneofficial
Twitter.com/@PositiveSue

MY WEBSITES:

Suestone.com
Suestonefoundation.com

1.
NEVER GIVE UP ON YOUR DREAMS

To think that years ago I had forgotten what it felt like to be happy! The thought of living a life I loved was totally out of the question.

I wrote about the first few years of my evolving journey in my book "Love Life, Live Life" and since then I've discovered so much more about myself and life, for which I am very grateful.

Along the way I have set many varied goals and observed with excitement and delight as they have manifested in my life. If I had let my analytical and logical mind take over, I would never have dared to dream that I could create a wonderful life for myself and my 3 children.

We all have this amazing limitless potential. Let's discover in this book how to tap into the infinite source of love, wisdom and guidance that is available to *every single one of us.*

Some people are born with faith and are wide awake to spiritual truth, others like I certainly was, have no memory or conscious awareness of any or very little of it.

3

Oh and how that led to my downfall. I've joked over the years that I've done everything badly, ever so well! However in truth, now I look back, I was fighting my corner and in the various crises that seemed to go on far too long, I really thought I did the best I could in the moment with all the knowledge, self-awareness and consciousness I had at the time.

Following my "wake up" call, I've consistently "worked" on myself, let go of the past and any negative and self limiting thoughts and beliefs, forgiven myself and others, embraced compassion and discovered self love; all hugely powerful if you wish to move forward, to live your best life and be true to who you really are.

In Love Life, Live Life I wrote the first chapter entitled "The Worst Year of My Life" and I certainly don't want to repeat it all here, but if you haven't read, heard or seen anything before here's an extremely brief and lighter resume of it!

In 1999 I was single (ish!), a soon to be divorced, mother of 3 young children left with huge debt following my marriage breakdown 2 years previously. I had the bank about to repossess my home, a collection of credit cards and loans, the odd bailiff turning up, a flashy car on high finance with negative equity and an on/off love at first sight relationship with a new man! I truly had forgotten what it felt like to be happy and I thought happiness had gone forever. I was consumed with desperation, negativity and fear.

Having been robbing Peter to pay Paul for some time, the turning point came when one day I realised I'd maxed out on every single bank account I had...the credit cards, overdrafts, loans etc and I couldn't get my hands on a single penny! I desperately grabbed my handbag and realised I had just £10 left in my purse and no idea where the next penny or few pounds would come from.

There was not an ounce of food in the house or petrol in the car. I knew I had to put £5 worth of petrol in the car for the school pick-up and I spent the rest on sausages and potatoes for the kids' supper. I hated to admit it then as I was SO embarrassed about how bad my life had become, but the rest went on the cheapest bottle of wine for me. Wine definitely helped numb the pain for me at the time as I was not aware of the "bigger picture" and any other self help and healing tools in that moment that I could tap into and use.

That £10 moment though was the turning point! My "wake-up" call as I now refer to it and the rest, as they say, is history! I made it my mission to work on myself and change my life. There's no point reading all the books, going on course after course and knowing what to do, we must do and be what we know!

I urge people to please not wait until you get as desperate as I was or for a crisis in your life, before you "wake up" and wholeheartedly embrace this way of living.

It is my intention that this book will inspire others to dare to dream and hold on to any vision with the knowing that we can all create a life we love, a life of inexpressible joy.

Years back it took me a while to realise that creating a dream life is an inside job. Once we create an inner world of peace, love, harmony and joy, our outer world reflects; in turn we are so much more empowered and equipped to help others around us and across the world, each of us in our own unique way.

In the following chapters I've explained very simply (as simple works for me!) what has helped me SO much at every level of my being; the rocket fuel for my mind, body and soul.

I believe if you embrace this way of being wholeheartedly and ignite the "blast off" tips and tools, you too can propel yourself into creating a life you love and beyond.

2.

"MY LIFE IS MY CREATION AND I CAN CHANGE IT"

When I woke up the following morning after I found I had just £10 left I cried and I cried. How on earth had my life come to this! I knew I had to take some practical steps, which I did baut it took a lot of courage at the time. I also came "clean" to a few close people who helped me out, giving me some cash or bringing boxes of food and wine around.

I remember thinking "Sue Stone if you don't do something to help yourself, no-one is going to do it for you!" It came to me that I must start reading and researching ways to change my life and that's exactly what I did.

In Love Life, Live Life I explained how I began to understand that there is a much bigger picture to life than the everyday challenges that we all face. I learnt about the power of our thoughts and feelings and about our conscious and subconscious minds and the universal laws that exist. I also learnt about the incredible power that is within every single one of us, and I have realised as time has gone by that so few people have any understanding of this power and have yet to develop and use it to its full potential.

Understanding and learning to consciously implement the power of our thoughts and emotions is a vital and necessary component to accomplishing and achieving a life of inner peace and joy and our most sought after dreams and goals.

The more I read and understood, I realised that it was me that had to make a major shift in my thinking and that the reason I was in my awful situation was that I had "attracted" (unconsciously) the situation in the first place! It was hard to take onboard at first but a lack of money or the fear of something going wrong was often in the back of my mind.

They always say "when the student is ready, the teacher appears" and since 2005 I've been working with tens of thousands of people across the world who, for whatever reason, have had their "wake-up" call or are simply looking for something to help them change their lives and circumstances for the better.

Often people have no conscious awareness (like me at the time) of how their life has got so bad! The "real truth" is that those circumstances are being created because that is what they are thinking or fearing at some level! The fact that they regularly think about what's negative or lacking is enough to allow the subconscious mind to begin the process of what it is designed to do; it absorbs the thought as truth, stores it and begins the process that will actually cause it to happen in the physical world.

When your thoughts are reinforced with emotions and words, it actually speeds up the process of materialisation.

This is scientifically proven and I'll share more about that later.

Many times, although they may consciously desire one outcome their predominant focus is placed on what they DON'T have or what they fear and as a result experience more of what they DON'T want.

What is crucial to understand is this. If you choose to have an abundant, happy and harmonious life, your predominant thoughts and emotions and the words you speak need to be focused on and in harmony with what it is you desire and NOT what is lacking.

We can dramatically improve the quality of our lives by taking control of our minds and manufacturing beliefs and expectations consistent with what we want to happen in the future.

Remember, you are what you think you are and you become what you say.

When you establish the belief that something will happen, the vibrational frequency of the power of thought, more specifically the emotion that these thoughts create and ignite, will attract precisely that which is believed.

"The universe is just a big Xerox machine. It simply produces multiple copies of your thoughts" Neale Donald Walsch

The thing about this is that everybody is always right! The negative thinkers say "I knew it would go wrong" or "I knew it wouldn't work" and the positive thinkers say "I knew I'd find a way" or "I knew the solution would present itself".

It's important to shift with lots of tiny steps into becoming "solution conscious" as opposed to "problem conscious", to being in a state of gratitude and love for the good in your life *right now*, however small it may appear, rather than being in a state of fear and lack.

It really does need to be a *moment by moment* awareness, especially in the beginning. Become the "observer" of yourself and ask yourself regularly throughout the day "What am I thinking? What am I feeling? And What am I saying?"

Remember, every thought you think, every emotion you have and every word you speak affects you at the energetic (quantum) level. (More about that later).

It's all about your state of "being" in the NOW, in this moment.

You do not attract what you want, but what you are!

The following statement is hugely powerful and well worth remembering to help keep you on track.

The way you FEEL in EVERY moment is what you are creating for your future

In *every* moment you are radiating energy (in fact you ARE energy) out into the universe and physics says your outgoing signal is *always* matched by the incoming one.

Remember every one of us today in this moment is the "product" of our previous programming, conditioning, experiences, culture etc and this is what makes up our consciousness, our energy field, our vibration.

Very simply put our consciousness is made up of;-

Our thoughts
our intentions
our feelings
our beliefs about ourselves and
our beliefs about life

These beliefs can be very positive ones or very negative ones, or something in between and very often borne out of what can appear to be very real "truths" at times. These are supported by your life experiences and in particular your programming as a child, which is a time when you were particularly open and would easily absorb the beliefs and attitudes of your parents, role models and teachers.

We often hear the phrase "Your perception is your reality". Albert Einstein said "Reality is merely an illusion, albeit a very persistent one".

The truth is that you are creating your reality of a world that surrounds you, a bubble of experience which accompanies you wherever you go.

The existence of these little individual worlds we all have, accounts for people having such different experiences even when they are in the same location. Some people perceive life as joyful, safe and loving, and others see it as dangerous and full of anger and hatred. If these are the qualities which dominate their consciousness, then this is what will permeate their bubble of reality and colour their experience.

Your bubble of reality is the focus of your life experience, the crucible or melting pot within which you create your own reality.

"Your personality creates your personal reality" Dr. Joe Dispenza.

If you haven't come across Dr. Joe Dispenza before, he is a scientist, neuroscientist, lecturer and author. He was one of the scientists featured in the award-winning film What the Bleep Do We Know which demonstrates a spiritual connection between quantum physics and consciousness.

So how do your beliefs affect your reality creation?

Your beliefs, especially those foundational beliefs which are called "core beliefs" become a key element in this whole process. A core belief has both an emotional and a mental aspect in it and that makes it quite different from any casual belief which you may happen to hold for a time, without any particular emotion attached to it, something that passes through your consciousness and is soon gone.

The dual nature of the emotional and mental aspect of a core belief reflects the way it emerges in your consciousness i.e. the level of emotion (energy in motion) behind the original thought, conscious or unconscious. A persistent thought moves through the stage of being a gut-feeling and finally settles down into a core belief.

A thought that goes over and over in your mind eventually gets accepted as a belief. This can work both ways don't forget, negatively as well as positively!

The energy in your consciousness is expressed as I mentioned above as thoughts, intentions, feelings and beliefs. All these, both conscious and unconscious, merge together to build your view of the world, i.e. your perception or picture of reality.

Your picture of reality is an important part of the mechanism by which you create your life experience.

Simply put.....

The thoughts, intentions, feelings and beliefs forming your picture of reality go out into the Universe as a signal, an instruction and this instruction attracts similar energies to you because like attracts like.

This is actually ancient wisdom that has been around since the beginning of time and in fairly recent times has been labelled the Law of Attraction. What I particularly love is that science is now able to measure and back up this ancient wisdom and I'll share more about that later.

Many people feel that they do not have the power to make major changes in their own lives and for that reason could not possibly be creating their own reality. What they don't realise is that their thoughts, intentions, feelings and beliefs simply provide the energy to send a signal out into the Universe. It is the Universe which amplifies this signal by adding all the energy required to rearrange a personal reality and manifest a new life experience.

The Universe links together the outer world of your experience with the inner world of your consciousness. The Universe is fluid and constantly rearranging itself within the bubble of your experience to create a reality that reflects your consciousness.

The Universe accepts what is in your consciousness without any attempt to edit or judge it. It accepts this as a symbol of what you wish to experience, your "home state of being" as it were, and it tries to reproduce this vibrational quality, this miniature "home" around you wherever you go.

So what is in your consciousness is the key to the whole process of reality creation.

If there is struggle and difficulty and suffering in your consciousness, then the Universe will reproduce all that around you, but if there is love, peace and abundance, the Universe will reproduce that instead.

Remember that it's a kind and loving Universe, God is a kind and loving God but the Universe is also an automatic system and it does not edit the contents of your consciousness. It does not say, "Oh, they don't really want THAT do they?" No, it just gets on and reproduces around you whatever happens to be in your consciousness. This is how the inner and outer worlds are linked.

Your outer world is a reflection of your inner world.

In modern Western cultures, people generally do not

see this connection between the inner and the outer worlds, so they tend to project judgement and blame outwards onto other people. They criticise and blame their partner, their children, their boss, their rival, their enemy, indeed anyone except themselves for the difficulties and disasters that befall them. And because they find it impossible to explain why some people enjoy health and wealth and others clearly do not, they rely upon the idea of chance or luck.

We've been conditioned to believe that we are separate from the world. If more people only knew that they have the power within them to shift their consciousness and that they are not weak, helpless and powerless victims of circumstances.

The following in italics is quoted from one of my favourite books, The Power of You, researched and written by my friend Ian Lawton.

"Every action in every moment within your reality you are projecting energy. There is not one moment within your reality that you are not outputting energy, and that energy that you are outputting precisely draws to you the same. You automatically draw the same energy that you project.

Close your eyes and visualise your body, standing.

Extending from your body is a shockwave of energy that is moving outward in the thrust, the intensity and the distance of a nuclear explosion in this moment.

That is how powerful your energy is!"

We are powerful co-creators!

There is a huge shift going on globally in people "waking up" and we're reaching a time in our history that many more are recognising that we are all a connected family on this planet and that we need to come together in co-operation.

Scientists have proved that EVERYTHING in our Universe fundamentally is ENERGY (More about that later).

What I find hugely exciting is that they have also proven mathematically that *every* cell in our universe is connected to *every* single other one! So when people say "We are all connected, we are all one", we actually are!

We hear the expression "I get good vibes about her or him" or you can walk into a room where 2 people have been arguing, even if they are not saying anything we pick up the bad vibes.

However, if I were to say that we are all "vibrations in nature" that could potentially sound a bit fluffy! But we are all a swirling ball of vibrating energy, consciousness (and we know from above what makes up our consciousness).

The key to remember here is that two things in vibrational resonance with each other are drawn together, that's science.

The indicator of the vibration you are on is the way you are *feeling*.

So if we think thoughts of what we don't want or what we are fearing, it's bound to make us *feel* negative and fearful and, quite effortlessly and often unconsciously, we draw more things to us to make us feel that way again.

Hence, as I mentioned earlier a hugely powerful and simple phrase to remember is "the way I *feel* in *every* moment is what I am creating for my future".

A negative thought only has power if you react to it and give it emotion.

It's OK to have a negative thought but remember not to feed it, it's like throwing fuel on the fire!

As soon as you start to live consciously and become the "observer" of yourself, you can very soon start to identify any self-limiting or negative thoughts and beliefs that you have that are contributing to the life you are creating.

Once you are aware of them, you are half way there!

Remember to convert your inner critic to be your inner coach.

As soon as you identify a negative thought that you are having, you have a choice on how you respond to it... I'll explain.

With me a huge trigger would be the arrival in the post of a threatening letter to pay a bill or Final Demand for payment. Once I started "working" on myself, I knew I had to consciously take control of how I responded to what was occurring.

So the choice I had.... I could either feed the inner critic, that self sabotaging voice in my head that could (and did at times!) turn it all into a "drama" in my mind.... oh no if I can't pay this, they'll send a bailiff in, everything will be taken, I'll lose my house, I'll be homeless with my children etc etc.... you get the drift.... and before I knew it I would be consumed with fear and negativity and of course the more I gave it emotion (energy in motion) the more I amplified the signal to the Universe to bring me more of the same!

So once I became aware of my negative thoughts around the letter, instead of feeding the inner critic I brought in my inner coach. How many people are brilliant at supporting their friends and being positive about their situation, encouraging them to stay strong, reassuring them they'll find a way, the solution is out there etc, yet when it comes to themselves totally forget to do the same!

The key is to acknowledge the "issue" to yourself, not suppress it as this can create dis-ease in your body which can manifest as disease, illness and potentially neurotic tendencies.

I would acknowledge the letter and say out loud to myself in a supporting way "It's ok Sue that you are having these thoughts and feelings because right now I have no idea how I am going to pay this. But I'm going to let you go negative thought as I am now open to all the ways money can show up in my life and I'm open to finding and seeing the solution".

Do you get my drift?

I *deliberately* shifted my thoughts to be "solution"

conscious and not "problem" conscious. I would also *deliberately* focus on all the things I had to be grateful for in my life right now and the people I loved. I consciously embraced the positive emotions of gratitude and love, a far more positive vibration to be radiating!

Remember, you get more of what you focus on!

We also have something in our brain called the Reticular Activating System. It's our own alert mechanism and our very own Google search engine.

I love this simple analogy and it often hits the message home with people who are more left brained.

If you were to key into the search bar of Google "failure, loneliness and poverty", for example, in a matter of seconds Google would bring to you right in front of your eyes millions of bits of information relating to "failure, loneliness and poverty".

However, if you were to key into the search bar "solutions, new opportunities and abundance" in a matter of seconds Google would bring to you right in front of your eyes millions of bits of information relating to "solutions, new opportunities and abundance".

Bearing that in mind, if I asked you to look around you right now and count how many things you can see that are red. Once you've done that, close your eyes and ask yourself how many things did you see that were green.

The chances are you didn't really notice the green, because your *focus* was on spotting the red!

This is what happens in life; if you constantly focus on the things that are NOT working, the things you DON'T want, the closed doors, the stop signs (red) that is all your brain will filter out for you to notice.

The green (the go signs) are all out there; the solutions, the opportunities, the perfect partner, happiness and abundance and so on.

Deliberately shift your focus to the "green" and be "solution" conscious and at every level you will be supported!

Please be aware that limitations are not imposed upon you, they flow from your own consciousness and are only valid and powerful when accepted by you. For example, if you believe that you must accept and live within your problems, then those problems become impossible for you to solve. But what is happening here is that your belief is stopping you from solving the problems.

"Each person is born with an infinite power, against which no earthly force is of the slightest significance." Neville Goddard

Through the core beliefs you hold in your consciousness, you are the author of your own happiness or your own misery. Your consciousness is a creative instrument of enormous power, but like any tool of great power, you need to treat it with respect and learn how best to use it.

As I mentioned above once you become the "observer" of yourself and aware of your core beliefs and you begin to change those thoughts and beliefs into something much more positive and more aligned with your aspirations and your dreams, the results can be dramatic.

Your conscious mind is equipped to examine both the outer world of your experience and your inner world of your psyche. As you begin to examine both these worlds, and compare them, your ability to change your reality consciously will increase.

Identify and weed out false beliefs and ideas that seem to be true, but are really not. A certain amount of detachment is needed for this process of exploring your core beliefs to be effective. In particular, you may need to become detached about your parents' or peers values and beliefs or anything related to previous programming and conditioning. Only then are you really free to construct beliefs of your own.

This process of self knowledge and awareness opens the channel to your own inner power and the rocket fuel for your mind, body and soul. Say to yourself "My life is my creation and I can change it".

Be aware of how big a step you have taken here since this is both a statement of empowerment and also a conscious realisation that you are in charge of your own life, and therefore, fully responsible for it.

You are now taking positive action to shift your consciousness, to free yourself from the chains of any limiting and negative beliefs. How exciting is that!

#BlastOffTips

We *all* have the seed of greatness within us, just like the oak tree is already in the acorn. With the right nourishing and nurturing it naturally emerges into its greatness; nourish and nurture you!

Become the observer of yourself and identify any negative and self-limiting thoughts, statements and beliefs that will prevent you from emerging into *your* greatness.

Work on 3 or 4 at a time that you wish to change. Stay conscious throughout the day and work on turning them round.

Deliberately choose positive and grateful thoughts, the thoughts that feel best.

What new positive thoughts do you wish to fire and wire? Just like the actor or actress does; rehearse and repeat them to install your new programming. Soon you will naturally start thinking, feeling and acting that way.

3.
ROCKET FUEL FOR YOUR MIND - QUANTUM PHYSICS MADE SIMPLE

Over the years of my continued research I have been fascinated to discover more and more about energy and the quantum world and how it backed up everything I was learning and applying from a more spiritual perspective. Both are intricately tied together and developing an understanding of them will arm you with an unshakable faith capable of manifesting dramatic and, in many cases, seemingly miraculous life changes in your life.

Although it is not necessary to have a deep understanding of quantum physics for our purposes, a basic understanding will assist you greatly in establishing the belief (faith) of how your life unfolds and supports what I have explained in Chapter 2. As a result it will enable you to further develop your ability to improve the overall quality of your life quickly and dramatically.

Quantum physics is the study of how, what and why everything that makes up the universe as well as everything in it, both the seen as well as the unseen, is derived. It is a detailed study of what is known as quantum mechanics, which determines how everything in the cosmos has come to exist, beginning at the atomic and sub-atomic levels. More simply put, it is an in-depth study of the building blocks of the universe.

Basically quantum physics consists of analysing things that are experienced in life in various forms and tracing them back to where they originated and were derived from i.e. energy.

I wish to keep this as simple as possible for my own sake as well as making it easy to understand for my readers. Of course if you are interested in taking it further I urge you to do your own research.

You may remember learning at school about Newtonian physics and how our universe was made up of solid objects, which were attracted towards each other by gravity. According to Newtonian physics, it was believed that atoms and the sub-atomic particles, of which they consisted, were of a solid nature.

What Albert Einstein and other scientists with their world-changing discoveries proved was that these atoms and the sub-atomic particles that formed them were not solid at all; they were, in fact, various frequencies of rapidly vibrating pure energy that gave them the "appearance" of being solid.

Everything that exists in the entire cosmos, which is experienced through the five physical senses, from the infinitely large to the infinitely small, from the macroscopic to the microscopic, went far beyond just the theory of trillions of solid atoms being attracted together by way of gravity.

Everything that exists, whether nature, sound, colours, oxygen, the wind, thoughts, emotions, the chair you are sitting in, your car, your physical body, the stars, your dog, your ability to see etc. exists only as a result of this very same energy.

To put it another way, ANYTHING and EVERYTHING that exists in the entire cosmos, when broken down and analysed into its purest form with sophisticated scientific tools and instruments, is merely a vibrating frequency of energy. This joins with energies of the same harmonious frequency or vibrational resonance as I touched on in Chapter 2 to form what we "perceive", and as a result experience in our physical world; our bubble of experience.

In the world of the quantum, science has found a world that is rich, complex and deeply intimate. Rather than a world of separateness and duality, it has found a world of oneness. Rather than a world of predictability, it has found a world of limitless potentiality.

Rather than a world that is merely here for us to use and enjoy, it has found a world in whose operation we are active participants by the mere existence of our consciousness - a world responsive to our awareness of it and our mental and emotional interactivity with it!

As I touched on previously we are not powerLESS victims in our Universe, we are powerFULL co-creators!

There is a famous experiment called the Double Slit Experiment and in essence this is what happened.

First of all remember that our universe is holographic in nature; a simple definition of a hologram is "the smallest part contains all the information that creates the whole".

For example, if you take a holographic 3 dimensional picture of an apple and cut it into 50 tiny pieces, you wouldn't have 50 tiny pieces of bits of an apple; you would have 50 tiny pictures of whole apples, albeit tiny ones, but every part of each holographic photograph contains all of the information that creates the whole.

Our universe works this way.

Atoms are the dividing line between Quantum Physics and Newtonian Physics. Another way of saying that is "tiny stuff", tinier than an atom and the "big stuff", bigger than an atom.

An atom is holographic in nature, it looks like a mini universe, just like the sun with planets revolving around it, an atom has a nucleus with electrons revolving around it. It looks just like our universe. The smallest part contains all the information that creates the whole!

So in the following experiment scientists said let's study these electrons.

They wanted to understand if an electron was a physical particle, a real thing like a marble or if it was a photon (a light frequency/wave length/energy).

They set up the experiment to specifically test for the physical particle and they observed that it was a physical particle.

Then they set up the experiment with the testing for the energy, for the photon... and they observed that it was a photon!

The important thing to understand here is you get

what you look for! It could be a physical particle or it could be a photon, depending upon how you frame it and what you are *expecting* to see.

The way that these subatomic particles behaved was influenced by the individual thoughts and beliefs of the scientist that was doing the observing. It wasn't until then that it was understood that these subatomic particles/waves/energy which make up everything that we can see and experience would literally change form into whatever the scientist who was studying it perceived and THOUGHT it to be!

In other words the energy being studied began taking form immediately based on the thoughts and beliefs of the scientist who was observing it!

The obvious conclusion they came to from this amazing sequence of events and experiments was that *everyone's* thoughts are also creative.

In other words this energy, comprised of these subatomic particles, is directly affected and takes form based on the thoughts and beliefs of the person thinking them. As discovered in the laboratories, this observed energy acts in exact proportion to the way that it is "believed" that it will act and will provide the physical appearance based on the "perception" of the thinker.

So to summarise, as our physical world is made up of atoms and electrons and our mind has the ability to influence them, then it's our thinking that changes the expression of our reality, and the more emotion attached to our thoughts amplifies its manifestation!

Wow wow wow! Don't you just love it!

Something else I found hugely fascinating and has really helped me expand my awareness and my belief that *anything* is possible is Non-Local Phenomena; Please do read on, I've done my best to explain it as simply as possible.

Another great example in Quantum Physics is called Non-Local Phenomena.

As I've just mentioned our physical world is made up of atoms and electrons; these electrons (sub-atomic particles) have a property called "spin". When two electrons are "paired", they behave as a single unit. If one spins up, the other spins down, if one spins right, the other spins left; if the spin of one electron changes, the spin of the other electron changes direction as well – instantly.

This famous mathematical "thought exercise" became known as the EPR Paradox put together by Albert Einstein and two of his associates, Boris

Podolsky and Nathan Rosen.

The exercise showed that according to quantum theory, this behaviour would remain unchanged *regardless of how far apart the electrons were from each other.*

They separated the electrons half way across the world and the very second they reversed the spin on one of them, the other one reversed its spin instantly. In other words, they would behave as one completely unified electron.

What this evidence shows us is the communication these electrons had were non linear; the distance didn't matter and time didn't matter.

When you bounce a football or a basketball you can see it bounce before the sounds comes to you, there's a slight delay because light and sound travel at different speeds.

However, what this is saying is there was no speed; the information was just everywhere, instantly, all the time, all knowing and omni present.

Very simply, no matter how far apart electrons are, they are part of an indivisible whole that cannot be broken into parts. There is no long distance communication; *there is an invisible and unbroken connectedness.* This Quantum Entanglement exists in the real world, but we can't see it. We can feel it, however, once the filament of connection is forged.

This was the first scientific proof of a web of connectedness between all things in the universe!

This is our intelligent Universe, God, Source and Infinite Divine Intelligence.

For those that may have a religious background, you will discover if you choose to delve deeply enough that what has been discovered by modern day science is precisely what the great spiritual teachers of the world have shared and attempted to get their followers to understand for thousands upon thousands of years.

The conclusions that have been arrived at thus far through the study of Quantum Physics aligns perfectly with what all the major religions of the world have always taught in some form.

Science and Theology are in fact closing in on each other. Science is saying that everything is energy and everything is vibrating. Everything has its own vibrational frequency. Science says energy is: "on the surface of universal consciousness which is omnipresent." Theology says, "God is everywhere – omnipresence".

The continuing studies can blow your mind away, every time scientists go looking for more, they find it! If you are interested in going deeper and further, I urge you to do your own research.

Please also note that there are still many different interpretations of quantum theory; what is for certain is that we will learn much more in the coming decades about the mechanics of how we create our own reality.

The fact that we are able to do it, however, is proven beyond doubt.

Every thought you think is heard by every cell in your body!

Have a read of this fascinating scientific experiment.

A gentleman was in a B29 bomber in World War 2 (where the gunner sits right out in the front in the glass bubble) and he agreed years later to be tested under laboratory conditions. They took a swab of the cells in his mouth and took this swab to another laboratory 9 miles away and observed the cells.

The scientists gave the gentleman a movie to watch of a B29 bomber in combat and the very second the bomber started firing right in a place where he would have been, the needle on the instrument that was monitoring the cells 9 miles away went crazy!

Evidence of non local phenomena; the cells were connected independently of time and space, instantaneous, everywhere, all knowing..... This is how your thoughts and emotions work!

Whilst not many of us have been in a B29 bomber, it's worth remembering that every cell in your body responds perfectly to every thought and emotion that you have. As mentioned above each cell is holographic in nature, i.e. the smallest part contains all the information that creates the whole.

This is one of the reasons why so many people have chronic health problems. How often do we hear people continually talk about what's wrong in or with their bodies? More on that in Chapter 11 Rocket Fuel for your Body – Living younger longer!

Different Frequencies or Vibrations

Think about this for just a moment. If everything in the universe is energy, then all that really matters is to understand that everything has a different frequency or different vibration. Let me share with you an example.

If we had an ice cube, we know that the ice cube is made up of molecules and atoms, two of hydrogen, one of oxygen, in a vibrational state that's called solid.

If we added some heat to the ice, then what we would be doing is speeding the rate of vibration and we would form a liquid. That's just a different frequency for the molecules.

If we were to continue heating up the water, then we would form something called steam. We still have the same proponents of water but it's now in a higher rate of vibration.

If you were then to continue increasing the heat to the steam you'd have gas or air. So it's the same molecules in a different vibration.

In our world, our language, we use things that we cannot see and we say that those are spiritual, they're in a spiritual vibratory rate. So what does that have to do with creating a life you love? Everything, because you are creating from the non-physical, the stuff you can't see, into things that you can see.

#BlastOffTips

Remind yourself regularly of this simple phrase that helped me so much years ago.

"My thoughts create my future".

Write it on post-it notes and place them where appropriate around your home and office.

What you think, feel and believe is at the core of who you are and what you create. Be mindful of what you are creating.

4.
WE ARE NOT HARDWIRED!

As I've already mentioned, there's an unseen world of infinite possibilities that we have access to.

However, we continuously live in the same reality over and over again, because we keep thinking the same way, we keep behaving the same way, we keep emotionally embracing the same feelings over and over again and that allows us to stay in a very predictable outcome.

If you carry on doing what you have always done, you will get more of what you have already got!

For years people have said to me "oh it's the way I am, it's in the genes, it's impossible to change" and so on and this ignited my passion to understand how the brain is evolving.

Neuroscience is the study of how the brain and mind work. In recent times neuroscience has taken a quantum leap in their theories and understandings proving that you *can* create new neural pathways and that we are not hardwired!

I think many people just get into the habit of

thinking negatively about their life. A habit is a redundant set of automatic unconscious thoughts, behaviours and emotions that is acquired through repetition.

The habit is formed when you have done something so many times that your body now knows how to do it better than your mind! Think about it, so many people wake up in the morning and they begin to think about their problems; those problems are circuits and memories in the brain. Each one of those memories are connected to people and things at certain times and places and as the brain is a record of the past, the moment they start their day they are already thinking in the past.

Each one of those memories has an emotion so the moment they recall those memories of their problems they feel unhappy, they feel sad and they feel pain.

As I have already covered, how you think and how you feel creates your state of being, so the person's entire state of being when they start their day is in the past.

"Your familiar past will sooner or later be your predictable future!" Dr. Joe Dispenza

I love Dr. Joe's way of explaining this...

"How many people do this I wonder.... they wake up, they grab their mobile phone or cell phone, they check their messages, they check their emails, they check facebook and they check the news. Now they feel really connected to everything that's known in their life and then they go through a series of routine behaviours. They get out of bed on the same side, they go to the toilet, they get a cup of tea or coffee, they take a shower and they get dressed. They drive to work the same way, they do the same things, they see the same people that push the same emotional buttons and that becomes the routine and it becomes like a programme".

95% of who we are by the time we're 35 years old is a memorised set of behaviours, emotional reactions, unconscious habits, hardwired attitudes, beliefs and perceptions that function like a computer programme and are automatic – driving a car, brushing our teeth, worrying about our future, judging others, complaining about our lives, not believing in ourselves, being chronically unhappy, just to name a few.

If you tell yourself just a few times a day I want to be healthy, I want to be happy, I want to be free and so on you are not going to get any positive change because the body is on a whole different programme.

Repetition is the key; this develops a new habit. In addition this is where meditation is of huge benefit, which I have explained in more depth later in this chapter and in Chapter 9. Through practice you can change your brainwaves, slow them down and enter the operating system. You can begin to make some really important changes.

Sadly many people wait for crisis or trauma to make up their mind to change and my message is why wait, especially once you discover how powerful this is. As Dr. Joe says you can learn and change in a state of pain and suffering or you can learn and change in a state of joy and inspiration.

I urge people to not wait until they get as desperate as I was and down to my last £10 consumed with unhappiness and fear until they "wake up" and realise just how powerful they truly are!

Often when people experience a traumatic event, they keep talking about it and reliving it (I was guilty of this!) and this has a knock-on effect. The stronger the emotional reaction you have to some experience in your life, the higher the emotional quotient. The more attention you pay to the cause of this in the moment, the brain puts all of its attention on the cause and takes a snapshot; that's called a memory, therefore long-term memories are created from very highly emotional experiences, negative and positive.

People *think* neurologically within the circuitry of that experience and they *feel* chemically within the boundaries of those emotions. When they have an emotional reaction or trigger to someone or something most people think that they can't control their emotional reaction.

I find this breakdown interesting.

If you allow that emotional reaction, it's called a refractory period. If you allow it to last for a few hours or days that's called a mood.

If you keep that same emotional reaction going on for weeks or months (for example, holding onto bitterness or negative emotion about something that happened months ago) that's called temperament and if you keep that same emotional reaction going on for years on end that's called a personality trait.

As I've discovered learning how to shorten your refractory period of emotional reactions is key and in Chapter 9 I've shared some powerful techniques that can help you with this.

When people hold onto negative emotion from the

past, what that means from a biological standpoint is that they haven't been able to change since that event. The emotions from the experience tend to give the body and the brain a rush of energy and people can unconsciously become addicted to the rush of those emotions. They use the problems and conditions in their life to reaffirm their limitations.

I can put my hand up and say that I was definitely caught in the "drama" of my life and all the "terrible" things that were happening years back, but I was totally unaware at the time of the impact it was having on my life; my mental, emotional and physical health, my relationships and what I was unconsciously creating.

Every time you recall the event you are producing the same chemistry in your brain and body as if the event is occurring, firing and wiring the same circuits and sending the same emotional signal to the body (and energetically into the universe to create more of the same!).

Remember, the same thought will lead to the same choice, which will lead to the same behaviour, which will create the same experience which produces the same emotion and so it goes on!

The key to change is not making the same choice as

you did the day before and that can at times feel uncomfortable in the beginning. Make the decision to live consciously and of course it all starts with your thoughts and where you put your focus.

The biggest way we can all maximise our brain potential is through the concept of focus or concentration. We have a piece of machinery in the brain called the frontal lobe. It's 41 % of our entire brain and the frontal lobe, to put it simply, is the CEO, the symphony leader, the boss, call it what you like and this is where our conscience resides.

It is what allows us to observe our actions, observe our thoughts, pay attention to our feelings and then decide on how we're going to change who we are to create a better life. The frontal lobe is connected to all other parts of the brain.

When we begin to use our forebrain in the proper way, we're inventing new possibilities, we're speculating new outcomes and we're paying attention by learning. When we begin to pay attention, the practice and art of paying attention allows the brain to move into more synchrony, into more balance and more coherence.

The opposite to that creative state is living in a state of survival or living in a state of stress. When we live in stress the exact opposite happens; we have the hindbrain now directing a forebrain and we live primarily by the emotions of the body. That's when people begin to develop diseases or begin to develop anxiety and depression because it is the chemicals of stress that knock the body out of balance, as well as the brain.

Just to be clear there is nothing wrong with having a short term stress response, we all react to the external world. The stress response is when your body is knocked out of balance but most organisms in nature are designed for short-term stress. It is when we start to have the long term stresses and the body struggles to recalibrate itself back to order that can potentially create dis-ease i.e. illness and disease.

Remember, what makes us so unique is that we can turn on the stress response just by thought alone and many people do it all day long!

What has been discovered over the years is that people are the most suggestible to the thoughts that are equal to their emotional state.

If they feel unworthy they will accept, believe and surrender to the thoughts equal to that emotional state and they will programme their autonomic nervous system into that destiny. This means they are less suggestible to the thoughts about empowerment and change if they are living in guilt, shame or unworthiness.

When a person deliberately changes their emotional state into gratitude and joy by focusing on the good in their life, they will more easily accept, believe and surrender to those thoughts equal to that emotional state. This, in turn, will programme their autonomic nervous system into a different destiny and scientists have measured the positive epigenetic changes (changes in gene expression) as a result of it.

Firing and wiring new neurons

So this is what happens.... simply....you think a new thought called I am healthy, I am happy, I am joyful, I'm in love with life etc. you signal a new set of neurons in your brain and you activate a new network of neurons.

You close your eyes, you begin the internal process and you begin to fire that thought but there's only one problem.... you've got all these other circuits firing at the same time.

In the midst of you firing this new thought called I am happy or I am joyful, you may well have all these other voices going on saying you're not very happy, you're a loser, you're too much like your mother or your father, you'll never change, look at you you're failing miserably here and what about the pain in your back!

Your inner critic or self-sabotaging voice is running wild! All of those voices are old circuits firing and wiring in your brain.

Now we have this amazing faculty as human beings, it's our will and our will is connected to our spirit. If you keep firing that thought over and over again (repetition, repetition, repetition!) and you keep firing it and you keep insisting that yes this *is* the thought you want in the front and centre stage of your mind. As you keep doing it, this will become the loudest voice and the loudest signal in your brain.

This thought I am joyful or I am grateful is now louder than these other voices and because this is the strongest signal the nerve cell has to wire to this one and glue itself together.

However, there's only a certain amount of glue to go around so it starts to "steal" the glue from the neighbouring circuits to connect this circuit and as it begins to connect this circuit it begins to disconnect the other circuits. That's because you are no longer paying attention to those thoughts!

As you continue to fire and wire, all of a sudden the only signal that's travelling to this neuron is called joy and gratitude. This in neuroscience is called "pruning" and this is exactly what happens in transformation.

The meadow analogy

I find this analogy really helps the understanding of the creation of new neural pathways

Imagine you have a big meadow with thick long grass ahead of you. You always walk down the right hand side of this meadow and the path is very defined. It's the path that everyone takes; this is our old negative thinking pathway.

But now, you are going to walk diagonally across the meadow, from the bottom right hand corner to the top left hand corner, it's a really sunny place over there! To begin with it is harder work making your way through the long grass; it feels strange and probably quite awkward as you are trying to create a new pathway.

If you were to walk that pathway once a day, of course the pathway would never become defined.

However if you were to walk that pathway many times a day, the more you practice it, the easier it becomes and the more quickly that pathway becomes defined. Repetition, repetition, repetition is key!

After no time at all it will be easy, the path will be totally defined and you won't have to put any effort into doing it, and that is what you are doing, creating new neural pathways in the brain.

Now think about this...... where every neuron connected to another neuron is called a memory, if those circuits are pruned apart then the memory of the old self literally no longer exists.

And where is that memory stored? In the soul as wisdom, how amazing is that!

Deliberately choose to be greater than your environment and deliberately choose to be greater than the conditions in your world.

What thoughts do you want to fire and wire in your brain?

What behaviours do you want to develop and demonstrate?

Along with your new positive and powerful self talk, visualise and rehearse these mentally, close your eyes and see and *feel* yourself living the abundant healthy life you would love to live with gratitude, joy, confidence and inner peace.

If you're truly present the brain does not know the difference between what you're imagining and what you're experiencing in the world. You then install the neurological hardware in your brain to look like the event has already occurred.

This means that your brain is no longer a record of the past, now it's a map to the future and if you keep doing it, priming it that way the hardware becomes a software programme and who knows you just may start acting like a happy person!

How meditation helps

Why is meditation such a great tool? When you sit down, drop your shoulders and close your eyes you are starting to disconnect from your outer environment. As you see fewer things, there is less stimulation going to the brain. If you're playing soft music or you have earplugs in, there is less sensory information feeding to your brain.

A clever tip I learnt from Dr. Joe when meditating is

to talk to your body as if it was a dog you were training. If you can sit your body down and tell it to stay like an animal, stay right here, I'm going to feed you when we're done or then you can get up and check your emails and texts etc but right now you're going to sit here and obey me!

I find just focusing on my breathe helps keep me in the present moment. If you find your attention wondering to a past event, which it probably will, realise that you are taking your energy out of the present moment into the past.

Settle yourself back down again into the present moment, just as you would training your dog and every time you do this, your will is becoming greater than the old programme you have been running.

Keep repeating this over and over again and every time you do this you are training and reconditioning your body to a new mind. (More on meditation in Chapter 9 Self Transformational Tools).

Neuroscience has measured this over and over again. It's exciting to know that, even when you think you are struggling to meditate and stay in the present moment and your mind wanders and you are telling yourself you can't do this, *every* time you observe those thoughts and take your attention away from them and back to your breath, you are making headway and in the process of change.

Every time you overcome just that one thought you are no longer firing and wiring the same circuits in your brain and you are no longer emotionally signalling the same genes in the same way. Slowly but surely you are liberating energy and freeing your body from the chains of the past.

When you begin to connect to source, when you truly surrender and allow your consciousness to merge with the greater consciousness, a loving intelligence and intelligent love, different compartments of your brain that were once divided begin to work together and synchronize.

When that occurs you start to feel whole, you start to feel more love for your life, you feel more spontaneous, more empowered, you feel clearer and you trust in the universe because your brain is now functioning in a holistic state.

You can't wait for success to feel empowered, you can't wait for your new relationship to feel loved or your healing to feel whole or wealth to feel abundant; that's the old model of reality, waiting for something outside of you to change how you feel inside.

The moment you start feeling whole, your healing begins and when you love yourself and you love and embrace all of life, you truly become a powerful co-creator and effortlessly create a life you love.

#BLASTOFFTIPS

Train your dog!

Don't get frustrated. Every little bit helps!

Day by day, inch by inch and it becomes a cinch

The more you love life *now*, life loves you back!

5.

So Why the Curveball?

There is something very important that you need to know and that is that it's not uncommon for a positive change in our lives to be preceded by a chaotic period in which a number of potentially unsettling things take place.

It's so important that you remember this because so often people are really working on themselves, changing their thinking, letting go of their past, focused on a fabulous future, being in a great energy in the now and suddenly this curve ball comes in and things can appear to be getting worse.

But this "getting worse" is often part of things getting better.

Of course "getting worse" may simply be that you are so negative that you are drawing more negativity to you.

However, if you have been working on yourself and have begun the mental and emotional process that allows positive change and seemingly impossible miracles to move into your life, often one can experience a clearing in consciousness.

This clearing in consciousness often results in the shifting around of many things and patterns in our lives. You may know this as "darkest before the dawn" or chemicalization but it is what is known in quantum physics as *chaos theory*.

In 1977 a Belgian chemist named Ilya Prigogine won the Nobel Prize for recognising that at the quantum level disorder can be the source of a new order.

In other words, a process takes place in which a quantum system reorganises at a higher level.

At a higher level that we as human beings are unable to "see" all we can "see" is the chaos or disruption going on around us in our everyday physical life.

For as we speak we are creating changes at the quantum level, as we think we are creating changes at the quantum level and as we imagine we are creating changes at the quantum level. We are reprogramming our consciousness and in turn our reality at the quantum level energetically.

In order for this to happen however, there is a breaking down in the existing system. This dissipation is essential to allow the system to reorganise and restructure.

Although the process appears to be chaotic, it is completely orderly and the system actually self-organises to a higher level of complexity and creates a shift in our consciousness.

Rest assured that the sudden appearance of order out of chaos is the rule rather than the exception.

This is an essential truth of the creative process. So remember the importance of chaos theory when you are working positively on yourself and perhaps trusting and praying or asking for a miracle and things seem to be going out of control.

It's very easy to become discouraged, angry or upset and to think and speak with great emotion during times of chaos. When you do this, of course, you are sending powerful but negative messages to the Universe.

Advice during Chaos Theory

No matter what is happening, stay focused on where you want to get to, stay focused on being very present in the Now, don't let your thoughts escalate out of control and certainly don't feed those negative thoughts and give them a load of emotion.

This is just the residue of your old consciousness,

your deepest darkest fears coming to the fore.

Those that understand chaos theory and spiritual law are undisturbed by appearance and ironically the best thing to do is celebrate, hold on to your vision and the key is to give thanks that the end is near and accomplished.

I understand you may have to deal with your inner critic, your self sabotaging voice. Let's call it Mr. (or Mrs.) Negative!

But remember Mr. Negative is fear; our own fear that we are not who we believe we are, that we do not deserve the good we have asked for. Mr. Negative wants you to stop planning for success and accept defeat.

Fortunately Mr. Negative is weak. He works hard, very hard, but he is not nearly as strong as your positive side. He can get you to make mistakes. He is full of logic and reason, hate and anger, jealousy and rage.

He is everything negative and desperate, but he is weak.

If you bring a lamp into a dark room, you get light. If you bring a bucket of darkness into a lighted room you still have light.

Mr. Negative is doomed to lose. He will lose because you have the unlimited power of the Universe at your fingertips.

So keep calm, take a deep breath and say out loud, "This too shall pass" "All is well".

These phrases I have used SO much in the past as I too experienced "chaos theory". Luckily I was aware of it and embraced it, but it can be hugely disempowering if you are unaware of it and have been consciously and positively "working" on yourself.

#BLASTOFFTIPS

Keeping your focus on your positive vision and remind yourself, again and again if necessary: Things are working *for* you, not *against* you.

Relax and trust that the Universe has your best interests at heart.

Remember, you provide the consciousness and the Universe, God, Source make it happen and find the perfect way.

6.
ROCKET FUEL FOR YOUR SOUL – FIFTH DIMENSIONAL LIVING

Embrace this chapter with an open mind, it may completely resonate with you right now or it may not! I wish to take this to a deeper more spiritual level which I have to be honest, some of it years ago I just didn't "get"!

Being conscious is the state of being aware. There are many levels of consciousness as they exist within the universe. Each level has its own natural laws and operates from its unique place within the whole.

What you understand in a particular way from one level of consciousness might look entirely different from another perspective. To be conscious is to know what is going on around you and in you and to see it for what it is.

To be spiritually conscious is to be aware of the Truth and to become free from the confines and limitations of the mind.

A shift of consciousness occurs, when we move from one level of experience to another. As we do that, we say "ah-ha", I get it; or now I understand. We can then describe our new insight from that level of reality.

As we make this shift in consciousness, the structure that holds the previous level in place must fall away so that the new structure can take its place. When this happens, we go through what could be called a "death" and rebirth experience, darkest before the dawn or Chaos Theory in Quantum Physics as I've talked about in the previous chapter.

Many are aware in these times that there is more than a usual shift in consciousness going on; a quantum leap. Astrology is helpful in explaining this phenomenon, as is Mayan, Egyptian and Native American traditions amongst others.

We are indeed going through a huge shift in consciousness. We as human beings are moving from a state of *self* consciousness to one of *unity* consciousness; from Third dimensional consciousness to Fifth dimensional consciousness.

Yes, Fifth Dimensional Unity Consciousness is here and you are living within it!

It is a "new world" based on moving from competition to co-operation, from control to compassion and from greed to sharing.

We are going through changes where we are beginning to understand consciously that there is no separate self but only unity in all things. I've already mentioned that science has proven that we are all connected energetically, that in itself is pretty amazing.

The implications of this shift in consciousness can be mind boggling for some!

So let me explain....

Just like we have different dimensions in this Universe, we also have different dimensional states of consciousness. These dimensions available to us on Earth are referred to as 3D, 4D and 5D.

These dimensions are not actual places but rather they are states of consciousness. Here on Earth, we are all living life in either 3D, 4D, 5D or a combination of all three.

In fact, it is most likely that the majority of people on Earth are moving back and forth across two or three of these dimensional states of consciousness depending on where they are in their lives.

Even though we are all living on the same planet and are surrounded by the same world, our perception of it will be different depending on which state of consciousness we are choosing to see things at.

Those perceiving things from a 3D state are going to walk through life much differently to someone perceiving things from a 5D state.

If you are curious what dimensional state your consciousness is at, here is a brief explanation of each:

Living from a 3D State

3D consciousness is viewing things from a purely physical state. You are seen as an individual that is separate from others.

Life feels like "the survival of the fittest" and you are identified by the way you look, the job you have, the car you drive and the people you surround yourself with. You may feel fearful about missing out or not having enough.

Things are perceived as being good or bad and life is a competition. There is not enough for everyone and some people have to miss out. Fulfilment is found in making money and social status.

You believe your thoughts have no power over your

reality and what comes your way in life is simply a coincidence. You rely on your five senses to move through the world.

There is a lot of joy in living life from the 3D state but pain and deeper emotions can be difficult to manage.

In a 3D state there is no desire to go within or to look at things from a deeper stand point. Life is played out by skimming the surface. There is no desire to dig deep or to understand the deeper meaning behind things.

Living from a 4D State

Many people believe that the 4th dimensional state acts like a "gateway" to the 5th. When in 4D it is easy to travel back to a 3D state, however this jump in consciousness is much more difficult when you reach a 5D state.

4D consciousness begins to awaken to the idea that we are all connected and that there is more to life than what meets the eye.

Thoughts are powerful and can shift the way reality is perceived. Duality and the idea of good and bad is still experienced, but there is more compassion and understanding behind it.

There is an opening to the importance of diet, meditation and leading a healthy lifestyle. What you put into your body becomes important and there is a desire to pay attention to how your actions affect the environment and those around you.

There is a strong desire to find your purpose and to follow your passions. You understand that life is meant to be enjoyed and that you are worthy to live the life of your dreams.

You perceive the world through 6 senses and your intuition starts to grow and expand. You seek a deeper meaning to life and you can start to see the synchronicity and magic of the Universe.

Living from a 5D State

Once you reach a 5D state of consciousness, it is very difficult to go back to a 3D state.

From this level of consciousness you begin to understand that we are all one and we are all connected. Life becomes an adventure of growth and there is no such thing as good or bad. There is a higher purpose for all things and every experience holds meaning.

There are stronger feelings of love and connectedness with others, the planet and even the galaxies around us. Love and compassion reign supreme and there is a lack of judgement. You understand that everyone is just on their own journey.

Everyone is considered to be equal and there is a desire to live from a place of pure authenticity. You understand that your purpose is to live your truth and to seek the joy.

From this state, you know that there is no competition and there is enough in the Universe for everyone. You feel overwhelming emotions of love and compassion for life, Mother Earth and the stars.

Your intuition is extremely strong and you feel connected to angelic and other dimensional beings/energies.

It is important to remember that these states of consciousness are not "better" or "worse" than the other.

Every soul on this Earth has their own journey to walk and their own reasons for choosing which dimensional state to live from.

I love this explanation from an angelic source called Alariel, channelled by my friends Stuart and Joanna when they asked for a comparison between third dimensional consciousness and fifth dimensional consciousness.

"5D consciousness is essentially lighter, clearer and able to see more options and think more creatively than the 3D consciousness. It is subtler, more attuned to the holistic totality of life and less involved with individual ambitions. It thinks of the highest good of all concerned, and not about personal advantage or the opportunity to acquire or gain.

The 3D consciousness of humanity is dominated by the hopes and fears and concerns of the personality in general and the ego in particular. The ego sees no life worth having beyond its own present state of awareness, and would like to lock you into this forever, but your essential nature works against this. You have transformation written into the very fabric of your being, and you are now entering a period of rapid change. Whether the ego likes it or not, change is inevitable and is happening all around you.

The result of this change will, over time totally alter your perspective and move you from a very limited view of life, a view imprisoned by the past, to one that is open to all possibilities. The most striking practical change will be the move from a competitive economy to a co-operative social structure, from greed and accumulation to compassion and sharing.

You're already seeing the beginning of this whenever a natural disaster hits a specific area of your planet At that point, you abandon the principles of competitive economy, one nation vying against another, and instead you act in a way that is not in your economic interest. You mobilize help from all over the world and pour money and resources and people and effort into trying to help the country which is suffering. So in times of crisis, you are already moving beyond the "greed and competition" scenario. When disaster strikes, you show that you understand the meaning of community in a global sense.

And it's exactly this sense of sharing and community that is now arising to save your planet from its over-competitive, consumerist nightmare. The materialist paradigm is now becoming recognised for what it is – both deeply flawed and divisive socially, and highly dangerous for the whole global environment.

Your science has also been evolving and your scientists are now discovering that consciousness and energy are not two separate things, but different aspects, different frequencies if you like, of one single thing. And the more powerful and developed a consciousness is, the stronger the energetic field of that person.

Here, it is a question of degree. The consciousness of the average human being is untrained, undisciplined and unfocused. It is like a diffused and weak form of light. The consciousness of a Master-soul is exactly the opposite; trained, disciplined and capable of a very exact and specific focus, like a laser beam. You can do very little with a broad and diffused beam of light, but you can do much more with a laser beam"

Very powerful and insightful, don't you think?

Typing this now it's taking me back to my "wake-up" call and oh my goodness was I heavily living in the third dimension! I was very much in survival mode and really couldn't think further than what was going on in my bubble of experience, my picture of reality that I had unconsciously created for myself!

I've heard the expression that you "move from survival to service" and looking back at my journey I can see how that started to unfold. I'm totally focused on the "bigger picture" now and the greater good for all but it has definitely been a process getting here.

As I said above these states of consciousness are not "better" or "worse" than the other. Every soul on this Earth has their own journey to walk and their own reasons for choosing which dimensional state to live from. However, with the way the transformational energies and vibrations are accelerating and rising, the lower denser vibrations are going to prove challenging to exist in.

Let's now cover this at a practical and grounded level...

Personal Empowerment – The Awakened Way, The art of living, loving and thriving in this new paradigm of the fifth dimension.

So what is it?

It's heart based intuitive living, not mental in the head living. The important difference here is to release the over analysing, the micro managing.

A hard one for many I know and that's been a huge shift for me. We have been conditioned and programmed in the old paradigm, shall we say the old operating system, that we have to "work it out" for ourselves, to take massive action consistently, it's a numbers game, you've got to work hard if you want to get anywhere and so on.

"The intuitive mind is a sacred gift and the rational mind is a faithful servant. We have created a society that honours the servant and has forgotten

the gift"

So true!

It's about "being" rather than "doing"; Tapping into the intuitive mind and working smart not hard.

Self love and self acceptance is also a big shift for many. Learn to love and accept yourself exactly as you are and if there are parts of you, behaviours etc that you don't like, do something about it.

Treat people as you wish to be treated at all times!

Don't start worrying that if you just accept where you are right now, you're never going to get anywhere else and nothing is going to get better, that's not true! When you just accept where you are and are grateful in this place, and appreciate that you are alive and breathing, you start to find your way in the smaller things, all the avenues of miracles and abundance, happiness and joy, open up for you.

That was a huge breakthrough for me, learning to live in the Now. Not resisting my situation, accepting it and deliberately choosing thoughts of gratitude and love, totally appreciating that THIS is the only moment I have.

We live in an eternal moment of NOW!

Remember your point of power is in the Now!

In this moment, right here, right now, at zero point, just you, your breath, this is where your power is. Not in the past with resentment, guilt and shame and not in the future with worry, anxiety and uncertainty.

This place of personal empowerment is a place of freedom and this is actually our natural default when we allow it to be so.

It's getting into flow and accessing the ability to give and receive equally; a lot of people are not in their empowerment because they don't know what it's like to receive or they don't feel worthy to receive.

You take yourself right out of personal empowerment and right out of an awakened way of living when you have expectations, judgements and attachments and when you are carrying others and they are not honouring their own journey.

When you start awakening and when you remember who you truly are, a perfect beautiful soul this creates new neural pathways which I've explained in Chapter 4.

This will *allow you to live in a default of thriving rather than a default of stress and anxiety* and, in the beginning, without any of the circumstances changing in your life whatsoever!

Nothing is outside of you, you are in charge of what your vibration and frequency expresses as you step into the awakened empowered way.

Instead of having to chase life, life will come to you, because your default is now to thrive.

If you are ready to step into your personal empowerment please read out loud, confidently and with positive emotion, this powerful Empowerment Prayer and visualise where guided to embed this energy.

Empowerment Prayer channelled from Archangel Gabriel

I AM myself

I accept myself

I value myself

I forgive myself

I bless myself

I express myself

I trust myself

I love myself

I empower myself

For all the times that I have given my power away to others or to fear,

I call that power back to me NOW

From this life or any other life, from this planet or any other planet, in this dimension or any other dimension … hidden or seen … I command my power back to me NOW.

Through every photon, atom, neutron and electron … through every piece of my soul fragment; through my higher soul portal, I call back all my divine, empowerment NOW.

So just visualise now…..

Visualise waves of golden and white energy coming to you …

breathe it in …

allow the golden light of your empowerment to penetrate your skin ... cocoon you in light and open your solar plexus.

Feel your power returning to you ...

breathe it in ...

Feel your personal empowerment ignite with every breath you take ...

Feel your multi-dimensional DNA activate ...

and feel the acupuncture points on your body fill with photon packages of light, assisting your DNA to remember your unique spiritual powers and innate abilities

Bask in your divine empowerment light.

Radiate your light back to the Universe and throughout the planet.

Proclaim from this moment forward ... say out loud or to yourself....

Nothing can dim the light that I shine from within.

I have ignited my personal empowerment ...

and now just breathe it in …

Feel your solar plexus open … you have called back all the power that you have ever given away …

And so it is …

thank you, thank you, thank you

It is done, it is done, it is done

(The End)

***

Wow, don't you think that is powerful? Do it every day if necessary.

You may find it easier to record it onto your phone in a soothing voice, allowing time for you to repeat the statements where necessary and so that you can guide yourself through the visualised sections.

This activation is an experience, so allow yourself to feel and truly experience it. The more you can experience the activations, the more of your latent and dormant DNA that is encoded within your empowerment activates. You don't have to do anything other than just BE a fifth dimensional being!

Claim it!

The Awakened way means you've got to have a lot of compassion for yourself, be kind to yourself and pick yourself up if you fall down. If anxiety comes up, allow it to be released, allow it to move through, don't wrestle it down to the ground and over analyse the you know what out of it, release it to source, to the angels, to God, to the light, let it go!

Be a witness, an observer, don't take anything personally! Don't take your inner critic personally, release your judgement on other people and then you don't need to take their behaviour personally, that's purely a construction of the ego.

Speak your truth from a lovely space. Communicate and work it out in a loving and compassionate manner.

A profound knowing will emerge once you awaken to who you truly are; that you are not broken and all that programming of being told blah blah blah as a child or perhaps more recently, means nothing now; nothing will tether you in the third dimension!

You don't need fixing!

Remind yourself you are on the road to

remembering who you truly are, an unlimited divine soul, a spiritual being having a human experience, a child of god, a goddess, whatever resonates with you!

When you can look at yourself as the Universe, God and your angels look at you, they do not see any character flaws! They see a divine beautiful soul.

People unfortunately put you into their reality, put you into a box, tether you, put you down, but that's what awakening is all about, releasing those tethers and chains so you can fly!

When you are in your personal empowerment, when you are living the awakened way you are free! It feels really good!

Any part of your life that you are trying to *make* happen in your life, that's third dimensional living; my value depends on it, my ego wants it so I'm going to get it!

If you're under pressure to get sales, to get leads and you are being pushed by your employers, for example, that's not feeling very fifth dimensional so reframe it!

Connect to your leads first energetically, reaching

out to their higher selves, what about meditating on who these perfect leads are and what energetic qualities they have. Meditate on how it feels in the heart (see also Five Steps to Access Your Hearts Intuitive Wisdom in Chapter 9 Self Transformational Tools) to connect with these leads and then take the *inspired* action, approach it spiritually, energetically, knowing that it is done and that everything happens FOR you not against you.

The inspired action then actually happens with ease and grace instead of running round like a headless chicken or a busy fool, doing a lot of things but not getting much done. There are too many people getting burnt out with stress in our society, their immune system shuts down and they lose clarity and focus and literally cannot see the wood for the trees. (Been there, done that!!)

Don't worry about mistakes, those "m" words are just course adjustments, they are purposeful and driving us somewhere, don't judge them as something bad.

Take away good and bad and call things colourful! It takes the sting out of it all! Remember to come from a place that everything happens FOR me. It's just redirection and refocus. Trust that the universe knows what the highest vibrational trajectory is for you but you've got to be in the space to allow that to happen. Do not wallow!

Reframe things in your life, call them colourful and find the silver lining, there is always a silver lining so don't give up until you find it! Ask your higher self, your guides and angels, something rather colourful has happened, please show me the silver lining! Keep invoking that and keep that awareness in your consciousness, being in the receiving mode and then you will start to see what's on the other side of what's happening.

Personal empowerment and stepping into your power, for some, can be a conscious fear and for many a subconscious one. It can create fear that your old life may change, have to collapse, that things won't resonate anymore and things will fall away.

Meditating, walking in nature and experiencing joy can shift that subconscious programming. Keep asking your higher self, the angels, God, (whatever is right for you) to show you and if you keep taking an honest assessment of patterns that keep re-occurring in your life, you will start to see where those subconscious programmings lie i.e. I'm not enough or I'm too much. Please remember you are just right as you are!

As I said earlier, be kind and compassionate to yourself. Don't over analyse, honour how you feel and allow it to shift through, relax and go with the flow. BE rather than DO.

The fifth dimensional portal is a space of pure potentiality, of infinite possibilities, limitlessness and miraculous healing.

The fifth dimensional portal has 2 passwords

Allow and surrender!

For some men especially and left brained ladies that can be really scary, I've had to work through that too.

The exciting thing is when you step into that Personal Empowerment you truly can create seemingly impossible miracles and abundance by *allowing and surrendering.*

Ask your higher self, your guides and angels to show you and, if you haven't already, develop the conscious connection between you and them.

Ask! Show me my plan or better! Better always shows up! BE open and in a state of allowance and trust.

Trust is so important. Many know the expression "Let go and let God". It's almost like you are floating on water, you just have to have that trust. It can be so hard for us as humans to trust in something that we cannot physically see, but we all breathe air, we can't see it but we are breathing it.

There is so much release if you can allow yourself just to BE in that energy of receiving, allowing and surrendering and asking your guides and angels to show you. It is so empowering to know that you can just BE here now, embody yourself now and stop extracting "stuff" from the past and your previous experiences.

In Chapter 9 Self Transformational Tools I share a wonderfully powerful mantra that will enable you to "clean" old memories, old data and live your life from inspiration rather than from memory.

Seriously, this shift for me has been huge; I used to over plan and have a need at some level to always be busy and in control.

For years now my main focus has been to embrace, love and thrive in the Now, as after all, it IS the only moment we have.

Every day I walk out in nature, tune in and say to the

higher powers that be "Show me if there is anything you wish me to do and I'll do it, nudge me, make it clear to me" or words to that effect. I have committed myself to love life, to work for the greater good of humanity, to help raise the vibration of our planet and I believe we *all* have our own *unique* part to play.

Just to conclude this chapter, I wish to share some wonderful words from Sadhguru, an Indian yogi, mystic and author.

"Be clear of what you want. Humans wish joy and peace and a loving world.

All humans are seeking pleasantness; Pleasantness within himself and pleasantness around him.

This pleasantness, if it happens in our body we call this health and well-being.

If it happens in our minds we call this peace and joy,

If it happens in our emotions we call this love and compassion and if it happens in our energy we call this bliss and ecstasy

Create yourself as a pleasant human being at all levels; peaceful, joyful and loving.

Commit yourself to creating a peaceful, joyful, loving world both for yourself and everybody around you.

For a committed man there is no such thing as failure. If you fall down 100 times, 100 lessons to be learnt. Commit yourself to creating a joyful, loving world in your thoughts and emotions and your energy will get organised in the same direction.

Once thought, emotion and energy are organised, your body will get organised. Once all four dimensions are organised in the same direction, your ability to create what you desire is phenomenal!

You are the creator!"

#BlastOffTips

Every morning set this intention; say it out loud with positive emotion. "Today everywhere I go I create a peaceful, joyful and loving world". We need to BE the change we wish to see in the world!

Remember, THIS moment right NOW is all you have got. Live consciously and monitor your energy, your state of BE-ing.

Train yourself to thrive in the Now and you will be perfectly aligned vibrationally and in the flow to create a life you love and beyond!

7.

The Key to Manifestation – Science and Spirituality Combined

Whilst I have covered significant areas and with the desire to reiterate and re-affirm what I have already written, I felt really inspired to write this chapter on the keys to manifestation; explaining simply how science is now catching up with ancient wisdom, the very ancient principles that have been here for 5-6000 years.

What it's doing is bringing together 2 great ways of knowing into a single wisdom; this can help us to become better people creating a better world, not only for ourselves, but with the right intention and collective co-operation and collaboration for the greater good of all.

For years we have been conditioned to believe that we are separate from the world and it is a matter of working hard and hoping for the best. However, we are reaching a time in our history where more and more recognise that we are all connected and that we do need to come together in co-operation, each of us with our unique part to play; not that we impose our will or control or manipulate our reality, that's not what this is all about.

Every single one of us has so much power within us to create great things in our lives, to create a life we love but I see many people often unaware and unconsciously NOT using the correct scientific and spiritual formula, for want of a better way of putting it.

Let me explain.....

New studies are showing that the human heart is the strongest biological generator of electrical and magnetic fields in the human body.

The brain has an electrical field and it does have a magnetic field, but they're relatively weak compared to the heart.

The reason this is important is that the physical world, as I've already explained, is made of those two fields of energy; electrical and magnetic fields of energy = electromagnetic fields.

Our own physics books now tell us if we can change either the magnetic field of an atom or the electrical field of the atom, we literally change that atom.

So if you want to change what is in your reality you have to change either the electrical field or the magnetic field, and there is a term for both, the stark effect and the Zeeman Effect.

(Johannes Stark 1913 German Physicist – Electrical fields, Pieter Zeeman 1896 first observed Dutch Physicist – Magnetic fields)

It's also telling us that when we have a *feeling* in our heart we are actually creating the electrical and magnetic waves that change the quality of the atoms of our world; they literally interrupt the flow of time and space and rearrange the "stuff", this world is made of.

Certain kinds of heart-based experiences such as appreciation, gratitude, forgiveness and compassion are the ancient understandings that have always been taught in the truest traditions of our past. Now our own science is finding that those same traditions are documenting this very real effect in our hearts.

The bottom line for all of us, and this is what the ancient wisdom and traditions always said, is that we are invited to *feel the feelings* in our hearts for the things we would like to experience in our lives *as if they have already happened*, rather than asking for them to happen and coming from a place of lack, of need and feeling powerless, which we have all done at times in our lives.

The 5000 year old texts left us very clear instructions that when you would like to change your world or change your body, rather than feeling what you don't have, feel as if it has already happened.

I talk about this a lot, it's not just our thoughts, it's the feeling associated with those thoughts. I can truly appreciate how challenging it can be to FEEL joy and happiness when things are going horribly wrong in your life.

How I dealt with it when I was desperate, and this was long before I knew about the science that backs this up, I had to get back to basics and deliberately focus on all the things I had to be grateful for, however small, and focused on the people I love.

Gratitude is the power cord to the universe.

When you get that feeling, that emotion of gratitude and love, as opposed to fear and desperation, (but remember either way it's always working), that feeling is creating the electrical and magnetic waves that speaks to the intelligent field of energy, the matrix in our universe that underlies our physical reality.

Our outgoing signal is always matched by the incoming.

Or very simply put.... and I say it again.....

The way you FEEL in EVERY moment is what you are creating for your future!

This is another reason why people do not achieve successful and rewarding manifestations. They do their affirmations, visualisations, meditations etc in the morning and the rest of the day get caught up in the drama and stress and frustrations of the day and their predominant energy they are emitting is stress and frustration, which creates more things to stress about and be frustrated with.

In Chapter 10 I cover more reasons why many do not achieve their desired results and how to fix it.

Some people do 100s of affirmations every day but an affirmation without emotion is an empty thought with no energy. This is why they lose interest, they become disempowered and say this stuff doesn't work, that's because they've only been using half of the formula.

This intelligent field of energy is a non conventional field of energy, it's not like electricity and it's only in relatively recent times that scientists and physicists have had wide spread access to the technology and equipment to measure it.

Thoughts are important but the new studies are showing that even though the human brain does create electrical and magnetic fields they are relatively weak compared to the heart.

The heart is about 100 times stronger electrically than the human brain but the heart is about 5000 times stronger magnetically than the brain.

So if we are going to create an electrical or magnetic field that affects our reality, it can be done with thought only but it is so much more difficult, it is much easier to feel the feeling with our hearts.

This gives power to our thoughts; a hugely powerful internal technology!

The feeling is the union of thought and emotion; the feeling is what creates the waves that "speak" to the field, the matrix in our universe. The thought is the image of the quantum possibility and in the realm of all possibilities everything already exists; the perfect relationship, the perfect job, perfect health and to bring it into this world and breathe life into that possibility, the power of human emotion, our love for that possibility, or fear, brings that into our reality.

So the key to successful manifestation of what you do desire is to practice cultivating that feeling, that vision and belief that it is already given even if it hasn't quite yet reached you in your today physical experience.

Give the field something positive to work with and then the field can give it back to you.

I promise you it's worth putting in the effort required in the beginning, and yes it does take practice, but look if I can do it, anyone can!

And as I'm always banging on, our point of power is in the NOW and with the 5D transformational energies in our universe accelerating, if we can thrive and be grateful for the good in our life right now, life effortlessly comes to us, rather than us having to chase life.

To conclude this chapter the following is a transcript from the angelic source Alariel, channelled by my friends Stuart and Joanna, which totally cements all of the above.

"Feeling and belief are keys to the creative process at all

levels. Creating comes from the heart, not from the head.

At any of the three levels, you can use your focus to create a reality, but that focus is most effective when free of ego and judgement.

Focus on the wish fulfilled, the outcome achieved, the reality created. In other words, focus on the experience of arrival at the destination and not upon the journey.

Feel into and experience as fully as you can the answer, the solution, the achievement; don't lock yourself into the question, the problem, the journey.

Enjoy the results rather than struggling with the process of achieving them.

This works at each of the three levels, the personality, the soul and the spirit (higher self) because by focusing in this way, you are aligning yourself with the universal web and the way the web creates reality.

Central to this creative process is a belief that this is really going to happen, but when that belief is strong enough to become faith, the whole process moves up a gear".

On the point of faith, I most certainly was not born with an unwavering faith in God or the Universe. This was something I had to work on.

Here are 2 of my very first affirmations once I became aware all those years ago.

I trust in the power and the magic of the universe

I believe in miracles, miracles happen to me

I repeated them over and over again throughout the day and we all know the benefits of repetition. A thought that continually goes through your mind eventually gets accepted as a belief.

From my perspective building my faith was a bit like compound interest, it starts small and builds and builds on the original.

Once you have an unwavering faith in place and surrender and allow the intelligence of God, Angels and our divine universe to work its magic, this is when seemingly impossible miracles occur in your life.

#BLASTOFFTIPS

Practice cultivating that feeling, that vision and belief that it is already given even if it hasn't quite yet reached you in your today physical experience.

Reach for the thought that feels best.

Give the field something positive to work with and then the field can give it back to you.

8.
MANIFESTING ABUNDANCE

Of all the challenges I went through years ago my biggest fear and that which created the greatest stress was lack of money.

Having been robbing Peter to pay Paul for some time, the turning point came, as I mentioned in Chapter 1, when one day I realised I had maxed out on every single bank account I had...the credit cards, overdrafts, loans etc and I couldn't get my hands on a single penny! I desperately grabbed my handbag and realised I had just £10 left in my purse and no idea where the next penny or few pounds would come from.

I remember thinking how on earth had my life got to this point! I was terrified but I knew at some level it was down to me. That set me on my road to discover and research ways to change my life.

I made it my mission to "work" on myself and with all the research I was doing, I soon realised I had to change my whole thinking around money and my attitude towards it.

Understand the purpose of money; what is money?

Money is one of the most emotional subjects on the planet and we put so much meaning onto it, yet the purpose of money is simply to allow the smooth exchange of goods and services!

First of all I wish to explain simply about the history of money because the more I've learnt about money and the banks, it really has put a whole new slant on money for me.

Let's go back a few thousand years when conch shells were exchanged as a form of barter. People literally "shelled out" in exchange for food or labour.

Then in the Roman times the mine workers were paid in salt or "salarium" which they could then exchange for goods and services. This is where the idea of working for a "salary" came in and the expression "worth your weight in salt".

As time went by and trade became more and more complex, the use of commodities like shells and salt were replaced by the use of precious metals.

Once trade became more centralized the direct exchange of precious metals was replaced by IOUs or Promises to pay.

Firstly they had coins as the officially sanctioned

IOUs followed fairly quickly by pieces of paper (bills of exchange/ promissory notes) that could be exchanged for precious metal.

In fact the pound got its name because until a few hundred years ago it could be exchanged for a pound-weight of sterling silver.

In the late 19th century an international system was set up called "the gold standard" which allowed for a universal and stable unit of valuation. Finally in the 1940s the governments of the world decided to abandon the gold standard system.

Promises of exchange were replaced by articles of faith, by that I mean the marketplace's faith that the government that printed it will continue to back it with or without reserves of gold.

In this sense money no longer has any intrinsic value. It's Fiat money that has been established as money, often by government regulation and only has value because a government maintains its value, or because parties engaging in exchange agree on its value.

Bank of England notes cost a few pence but what gives them value is purely the "trust" and "faith" and the confidence in its value. The value of money is now based entirely on the value we and others place upon it.

Have a read of this short story about a little Greek village. It really helped me years ago shift my thinking around money.

It is a slow day in a little Greek Village. The rain is beating down and the streets are deserted.

Times are tough, everybody is in debt, and everybody lives on credit.

On this particular day a rich German tourist is driving through the village, stops at the local hotel and lays a €100 note on the desk, telling the hotel owner he wants to inspect the rooms upstairs in order to pick one to spend the night.

The owner gives him some keys and, as soon as the visitor has walked upstairs, the hotelier grabs the €100 note and runs next door to pay his debt to the butcher.

The butcher takes the €100 note and runs down the street to repay his debt to the pig farmer. The pig farmer takes the €100 note and heads off to pay his bill at the supplier of feed and fuel.

The guy at the Farmers' Co-op takes the €100 note and

runs to pay his drinks bill at the tavern. The publican slips the money along to the local prostitute drinking at the bar, who has also been facing hard times and has had to offer him "services" on credit. The hooker then rushes to the hotel and pays off her room bill to the hotel owner with the €100 note.

The hotel proprietor then places the €100 note back on the counter so the rich traveller will not suspect anything. At that moment the traveller comes down the stairs, picks up the €100 note, states that the rooms are not satisfactory, pockets the money and leaves town.

No one produced anything. No one earned anything.

However, the whole village is now out of debt and looking to the future with a lot more optimism!

Just like that!

Have you heard of or got your head around "cryptocurrency" yet? I wouldn't blame you for a minute if you hadn't - all that technical jargon is enough to put many people off.

However, I feel cryptocurrency is certainly one signal that reflects a mobile shift of resources and energy from the old world, 3D consciousness and towards more 5D consciousness as I've written about in Chapter 6.

We are at the birth of a new revolution in the way we transact and consume within society. Just as in the 1990's the internet delivered a profound quantum shift in the way people can communicate and connect, so cryptocurrency has the capacity to unravel the very bedrock of the old banking system of control.

Essentially cryptocurrency is a widely distributed digital ledger, based on highly advanced "blockchain" technology.

Put simply, you can readily create a virtual "wallet", pay value into it, which then updates across a distributed global system, which is (pretty much) totally anonymous and outside of the banking system.

You're then able to agree the cost of goods with a vendor, and process the transaction, without exchange or bank fees, at lightning speed. Currently there is an exponential growth of vendors out there keen to transact goods and services via some form of cryptocurrency.

It's clear to me, at the time of publishing this book that we are at the very birth of an exciting new wave of transacting, outside of the defunct, old world system. Yes, the old system will try to control it, but new crypto technologies are birthing day by day and this reflects very well the birthing of a new consciousness on planet earth and I would encourage you to explore it.

***

Attracting money is like any other skill set, you don't need to stop being yourself in order to learn it; you just need to open your mind to thinking about your life in brand new ways.

Money certainly doesn't buy happiness but I remember only too well that terrifying feeling and the worry of not having enough.

Of course financial freedom for one person might be quite different to financial freedom for another, depending on their lifestyle; however there is absolutely nothing wrong in enjoying lovely things around you and feeling abundant once you get your "inner" world right and not looking "out" there in the material world for your source of happiness.

There have been many studies around money and I want to refer now to Napoleon Hill's book Think and Grow Rich, which helped me hugely years ago.

He spent 20 years interviewing over 500 of the richest people and discovered that, without fail, they had followed the same simple blueprint for wealth.

All wealth is created with the human mind.... It is how we think, how we feel and what we focus on.

Poor thinkers will never be rich.

"Rich thinkers" will be rich regardless of the current size of their bank balance. Their attitude and mindset causes them to focus on abundance. They will naturally be noticing possibilities and living life on their terms.

If they are temporarily low on cash they won't be for long and they somehow always seem to find a way to do what they really want to do in their lives.

"Poor thinkers" on the other hand *want* more money; they feel they *need* more money. Their focus is more on what they're lacking; the things they can't afford to buy and even worse, feel resentful towards people who are already wealthy.

"Poor thinkers" even if they have big houses and cars are always filled with fears about the future and tend to have a mistrust of those around them.

However, if you are not feeling rich yet, don't worry; it's just an indication that your current wealth programming isn't as good as it can be! Your mind is like a computer and like a computer, it's only as effective as the software it's running.

From a scientific and spiritual perspective it's our consciousness, our energy field, our thoughts, feeling and beliefs around money, that create how we *feel* about being "rich" and being abundant and how we "see" our world and what we create as our reality.

So the big question! Do you have a poverty consciousness or do you have a prosperity consciousness?

Is your general focus on lack or abundance? Don't worry if it is on lack because actually the majority of people unfortunately DO have this mindset, I know I did and you CAN turn it round starting today!

All you need is the willingness to start thinking in a different way and the courage to take actions based on this new way of thinking.

I had to find a lot of courage from within me; it was either lose everything or feel the fear and do it anyway!

I've already covered why our thoughts, emotions and beliefs are so powerful and of course the same applies to abundance and money.

Be mindful too of what you are picturing in your imagination, what you are visualising.

"Your imagination is your preview of life's coming attractions." Albert Einstein

Visualisation is the most powerful single capability that we have as a human being and what people tend to do is visualise what they *don't* want to happen.

I was the "expert" at doing it all wrong!

I would actually visualise myself and my children on the streets, homeless.

I constantly thought about bills, how was I going to pay them, all the creditors ringing up the whole time and what was I going to say to them, will I be able to feed my children and so on.

The more we think, the more we visualise and the more drama we build up, the more fear we feel; before we know it we are paralysed with fear. We become more stressed, our immune system shuts down and we lose clarity and focus. We can't see the wood for the trees, i.e. we can't *"see"* the solution and our subconscious mind accepts it as an instruction and proceeds to manifest more of what we tell it...more lack and more problems!

A little book I found helpful is The Message of a Master by John McDonald. He talks about the inner mind and the outer mind, the subconscious and the conscious.

He talks about how the inner mind is the one with all the power and its natural state is abundance; however why things go wrong is that, when one is not living consciously and being mindful, the outer mind (conscious thinking mind) judges everything by what the eye and the ear report. It transmits those messages to the inner mind (subconscious mind); what we see and what we hear gets accepted by the subconscious as our "truth". This "truth" manifests and becomes our reality.

As we know everything in our universe is energy.....including money.... and negative thoughts, emotions and beliefs around money are effectively creating a resistance to your flow of money.

By thinking happy and grateful thoughts, you feel happier and grateful and you will attract reasons to be happy and grateful.

To be rich, think abundant and grateful thoughts.

The *emotion* behind your thoughts amplifies your outgoing signal to the universe, which is always matched by the incoming.

The most important aspect of manifesting money is to approach it from the right heartset. Think of your heartset as the overall vibration of your relationship to the activity of attracting money. How would you describe that relationship? Is it greedy, needy, excited, hopeful, etc?

If you approach this process from a place of neediness, clinginess, scarcity etc you'll most likely fail. That's the right vibration for attracting nothing, or for making things worse by attracting unwanted expenses, but it's not the right vibration for attracting money.

If you come at this from a place of saying, "I really *need* £1000 or $1000 to pay my rent next month", if you focus on the need and try too hard you will create resistance.

A better vibration is that of hope, but this is still a pretty weak vibration.

A much better vibration is to come from a place of curiosity and experimentation. Get into a state of childlike wonder if you can, I appreciate that can take a little bit of "working" on when you are fearful, but it will definitely shift your vibe and create more positive results.

An even stronger vibration is to generate feelings of gratitude, playfulness and excitement. This is a great vibration for manifesting money. Train yourself to anticipate exciting things coming into your life, I found that really helped me hugely.

The highest vibration for attracting wealth is to feel rich and abundant now whatever your bank balance!

When you want to manifest money, it's important to know that it's already there. If it's hidden at all, it's hiding in plain sight, waiting for you to notice it.

If you think about it there are *vast* amounts of money in our world but it's just not coming into your physical experience. If it is lacking in *your* "world" right now, quite simply you are not vibrationally aligned.

Know that the money and the opportunities are right in front of your face. You just have to adjust your "eyes" to see them by shifting your vibration as above and your frequencies of thought and emotion to one that's capable of detecting and aligning with abundance and money.

So combining science and spirituality it's fun to think of this vibe-shifting process as shifting dimensions, as if you're tuning in to a different perceptual frequency spectrum. That other reality was there all along. You just couldn't see it before because you were tuned in to incompatible perceptual frequencies, frequencies that made the money invisible and undetectable by your senses.

Obviously your senses pick up a lot as you go about your day, but you only notice a tiny fraction of all that input. In order to manifest money, you need to tune your senses to bring to your attention useful input that you've been subconsciously dismissing as irrelevant background noise. This tuning process can take a bit of time and effort, but you can definitely do it. If I can do it, so can you!

Identify your limiting beliefs around money

It's all very well trying to shift your vibration, but where the problem lies for many is that they have been thinking their old way of thinking for such a long time and this develops ingrained limiting beliefs that so often people are completely unaware of.

They "normalise" a negative way of living, one focused on lack and limitation.

So first of all what you need to do is work on identifying any negative and limiting beliefs around money that are holding you back, and further on in this chapter I've shared some further useful exercises and tools to enable you to create an abundant mindset and a prosperity consciousness.

Consider and answer these questions..... jot your answers down.

1. What were you told about money when you were a child?

2. What did money mean to you as you were growing up?

3. What is your favourite saying about money?

4. What comes to your mind when you hear or read about wealthy people?

5. How do you feel about money now?

It's necessary to become consciously aware of your thoughts and statements around money. Be the "observer" of your thoughts and words....do you say or think any of the following?

Money doesn't grow on trees

There is never enough

I can't afford it

I am broke

Only the rich get richer and the poor get poorer

Filthy rich

Money is the route of all evil

Or any other limiting or negative statements around money.

If you *believe* you have to work hard for money or money is hard to come by you will only create a situation that you do have to work hard for money!

If you *believe* everyone is out to rip you off you will unconsciously attract people into your life that will do just that.

Whatever negative story you have told yourself in the past, it's time to let it go!

Just becoming conscious of your old programming around money is often enough to take away its power. So being "aware", being conscious is already creating a shift.

A really powerful exercise for you to do now that you have identified any negative or self-limiting beliefs is to write the following on a bit of paper and then burn it, setting the intention to release those beliefs holding you back.

"I am now letting go of my old beliefs that...(you insert as necessary)......as these beliefs serves me no purpose"

Obviously the burning needs to be done outside safely somewhere and when you are ready, read out loud your "letting go" statement. Say it with intention and conviction and then burn it. You may be thinking that it's a bit wacky, but trust me on this, it's powerful!

Give your mind new instructions and set a new intention to the universe

Now you've identified and set the intention to let go

of old beliefs holding you back it's important to ensure you don't use the old limiting language and thinking to re-create the same problem.

You do this by changing your self talk, which can so often be destructive. Remember you are not hard wired and a new thought that goes over and over in your mind eventually gets accepted as a belief.

Repetition, repetition, repetition. If you wish to be good at anything you have to practice and train, it's the same with your mind. It gets easier and easier I promise!

For fastest results have *a moment by moment* awareness of what you are thinking, what you are saying and how you are feeling.

Language like I am broke, I am frustrated, I barely get by each week etc must leave your thoughts and vocabulary!

A simple and effective way to deal with negative thoughts

I know I'm repeating myself here but it's important, so to reiterate what I've explained in Chapter 2.

As soon as you identify a negative thought that you

are having, you have a choice on how you respond to it... I'll explain.

With me a huge trigger would be the arrival in the post of a threatening letter to pay a bill or Final Demand for payment. Once I started "working" on myself, I knew I had to consciously take control of how I responded to what was occurring.

So the choice I had.... I could either feed the inner critic, that self sabotaging voice in my head that could (and did at times!) turn it all into a "drama" in my mind....oh no if I can't pay this, they'll send a bailiff in, everything will be taken, I'll lose my house, I'll be homeless with my children etc etc....you get the drift.... and before I knew it I would be consumed with fear and negativity and of course the more I gave it emotion (energy in motion) the more I amplified the signal to the Universe to bring me more of the same!

Convert your inner critic to be your inner coach

So once I became aware of my negative thoughts around the letter, instead of feeding the inner critic I brought in my inner coach. How many people are brilliant at supporting their friends and being positive about their situation, encouraging them to stay strong, reassuring them they'll find a way, the solution is out there etc, yet when it comes to themselves totally forget to do the same!

The key is to acknowledge the "issue" to yourself, not suppress it as this can create dis-ease in your body which can manifest as disease, illness and potentially neurotic tendencies.

I would acknowledge the letter and say out loud to myself in a supporting way 'It's ok Sue that you are having these thoughts and feelings because right now I have no idea how I am going to pay this. But I'm going to let you go negative thought as I am now open to all the ways money can show up in my life and I'm open to finding and seeing the solution'.

I *deliberately* shifted my thoughts to be "solution" conscious and not "problem" conscious. I would also *deliberately* focus on all the things I had to be grateful for in my life right now and the people I loved. I consciously embraced the positive emotions of gratitude and love, a far more powerful vibration to be radiating!

A negative thought only has power if you react to it and give it emotion

Remember *this* moment is all you have got and the way you *feel* in *every* moment is what you are creating for your future.

Abundance manifesting positive self talk and affirmations

Repeat out loud with positive emotion throughout your day any of the following that resonate with you.

I am open and ready to all the ways money can show up in my life.

Money is flowing to me from expected and unexpected sources.

Every day I am attracting and acting upon money making opportunities in my life.

I am activating my wealth gene and vibration to allow abundance and money to flow into my life.

I open to the flow of great abundance in all areas of my life.

Today I expand my awareness of the abundance all around me.

My grateful heart is a magnet that consistently attracts more of what I desire.

As my commitment to help others grow, so does my wealth.

Releasing every thought of lack from my mind, I now gratefully accept the abundance of good the universe has for me and I share it lovingly.

My day is filled with limitless potential in joy, abundance and love.

I am so happy and grateful now that money comes to me in increasing quantities through multiple sources on a continuous basis
(I discovered and used this one from Bob Proctor)

I do wonderful work, in a wonderful way,
I give wonderful service for wonderful pay.
(The subconscious loves a rhyme, thanks to Dr. Joseph Murphy for this one)

My own personal favourite at the time of writing this book...

I am rich beyond my wildest dreams, I am, I am, I am.
I am rich beyond my wildest dreams in love and joy and health and wealth.
Thank you, thank you, thank you

How to further shift your consciousness and

mindset to one of abundance and riches.

Deliberately make a point of noticing the abundance that surrounds you.

Train yourself to turn your attention away from anything that distracts you from focusing on creating wealth and well being. Of course that doesn't mean hiding your bills and refusing to face reality!

A good rule is…

Do what you can to improve the situation, then immediately move on to more positive pursuits. Just don't give the negative too much energy and worry about things you can't control.

Keep focused on where you want to be, not where you don't want to be. I cannot stress the importance of this too much! Hold your vision. Visualise and feel the emotion of abundance, success and gratitude as if already achieved.

It's a "win win" as the brain cannot tell the difference between what it sees in your imagination and what it sees in "real" life. In addition the feeling of abundance and success will align you perfectly for manifesting just that!

Our attitude towards money is vital too; be grateful for the money you do have and value every penny that comes in. Love it, appreciate it and value it!

If you get paid £100 or $100, rather than think oh that won't go far, think about the things that you *can* buy with it. It will increase the perceived value of the money you have in your wallet or purse. Your whole physiology, your body posture and your vibration will change.

Treat yourself to something, however small. Periodically I used to buy a cheap bottle of champagne, even when money was tight and I toasted life; for me it signified celebration, a prosperity consciousness and certainly raised my vibration.

Start saving 10p, £1 or £10 per week; this creates a new trend and pattern and sets a positive accumulative intention to the universe.

Love receiving and paying bills and be grateful for the service you have received. That's a big change of attitude for many; it certainly was for me in the beginning and took a bit of working on!

Clear the clutter – mentally, emotionally and physically.

"Your mind can be likened to a house that has been cluttered over the years with thousands of unnecessary pieces of furniture, pictures, ornaments, and other things, all strewn around and piled everywhere. The result is that, although the outside of the house may present a good appearance, the inside is a mess of confusion and disorder. It is impossible to accomplish anything under such conditions, for you cannot go after one thing without stumbling over another. There is no order. No purpose. No progress. The first necessary thing to do, then, is to rid that house of all but the furnishings that are essential to your success" Quote from The Message of a Master

In Feng Shui they look at the energy of a home and how it flows from room to room. When there is clutter in the home, it slows down the energy.

Money is energy: If you wish to have more money, you need to create space for it.

"When the magnet does not attract the needle, the fault lies in the dirt that covers up the needle" Sai Baba

If you live in your home surrounded by clutter and old papers it can be an overwhelming thought to clear it..... set a goal to spend even 10 minutes a day clearing the old to make way for the new.

Create a Vision Board and mock up a bank statement.

Visualise and feel how amazing you are going to feel with that amount of money in your account! Financial freedom, yay!

Remember the emotion behind the thought is the most powerful manifesting tool you have, but it works both ways. If looking at your vision board and bank statement creates any form of negative emotion, such as frustration or jealousy, this will NOT do a positive job for you. Only do this if it creates an excited and positive emotion.

Don't judge your future results on your previous experiences. If your financial situation and/or your business has or is creating stress for you Ho'oponopono it! You may well be wondering what Ho'oponopono is; I've covered this in Chapter 9 Self Transformational Tools)

Develop multiple streams of income, including passive income.

"Sit" or meditate for ideas. Find a way to use your interests and talents to contribute value to the world.

Identify a problem and become or create the solution.

Don't let temporary setbacks or defeats become permanent failure.

Successful people don't "do" failure, they call it feedback.

Successful people don't give up. They have passion, they have faith and they persist!

They understand the importance of patience and don't expect overnight success. Sow the seeds, nurture them and allow them time to grow, just like the arable farmer with his crops; he understands the laws of nature and the universe.

Punch the sky with success. Normally we punch the sky only when we achieve something great. Do this *before*, visualising your desired successful outcome as if you have already achieved your goal. Try it; you'll immediately radiate a success vibration.

The more you value yourself, the more the universe will value you!

I often share this when I'm speaking at events.

Some years back a speaker started his seminar by holding up a £20 note in a room of 200 people.

He asked, "Who would like this £20 note?"

Hands started going up.

He said, "I am going to give this £20 to one of you, but first, let me do this", and he proceeded to crumple up the £20 note.

He then asked, "Who still wants it?"

Still the hands went up in the air.

"Well", he replied, "What if I do this?" and he dropped it on the ground and started to grind it into the floor with his shoe. He picked it up, now crumpled and dirty.

"Now, who still wants it?"

Still the hands went into the air.

"How come you still want it?" he asked.

"It is still worth £20", came the answer.

"Then, my friends, we have all learned a very valuable lesson", said the speaker, "No matter what I did to the money, you still wanted it because it did not decrease in

value. It is still worth £20."

"Many times in our lives" he continued, "We are dropped, crumpled, and ground into the dirt by the decisions we make and the circumstances that come our way. We feel as though we are worthless.

But no matter what has happened or what will happen, you will never lose your value.

The worth of our lives comes not in what we do or who we know, but by who we are."

Please remember you are deserving and worthy!

Self love is a must and as you increase your self love and self worth, observe how your net worth increases.

The universe only gives us what we think and believe we are worthy of receiving.

On the subject of love.... learn and grow to love money! Most of us are conditioned to believe it's wrong to love money, but the more you can love money, the more it will flow beautifully to you.

Just think of all the good you can do in the world. Thank you, thank you, thank you!

Before I conclude this chapter on Manifesting Abundance, below are a Manifestation Oath and Prosperity Prayer.

As always I only share what has helped me so much. If either one or both resonate with you, simply say these out loud with positive emotion each day as part of your daily routine.

Manifestation Oath

"I accept and receive unexpected good, unexpected money, unexpected love, unexpected kindness, unexpected generosity, unexpected offers, unexpected prosperity coming in unexpected ways from unexpected places in my life and the life of others.

I am constantly guided, and boldly empowered, to receive the lavish abundance of the Universe!

I accept the Principle that abundance and prosperity have already been given to me.

My acceptance makes it real and opens the space for manifestation to rush in! I open wide the doors of my consciousness to receive and to give! It IS done now!"

Prosperity Prayer

Simply read it aloud with positive emotion every day for 40 days or longer if you feel you would like to.

"I am the source of all wealth. I am rich with creative ideas.

My mind abounds with new, original, inspired thoughts.

What I have to offer is unique and the world desires it.

My value is beyond reckoning. What the world needs and desires, I am ready to produce and give.

What the world needs and desires, I recognise and fulfil.

The bounty of my mind is without hindrance or limit.

Nothing can stand in the way of my inspired creativeness.

The over-flowing power of source energy overcomes every obstacle and pours out into the world, blessing and prospering everyone and everything through me.

I radiate love,
I radiate blessings,
I radiate creativity,
I radiate prosperity,
I radiate loving service.
I radiate joy, love, freedom,
health, beauty, peace,
wisdom and power.

Humanity seeks me and rewards me. I am valued in the world.

I am appreciated. What I have to offer is greatly desired. What I have to offer brings a rich reward.

Through my vision the world is blessed.

Through my clear thinking and steadfast purpose, wonderful new values come into expression.

My vision is the vision for the greater good of all.

My faith is as the faith of the undefeatable.

My power to accomplish is unlimited.

I, in my uttermost source, am all wealth, all love, all

health, all power, all productivity and all freedom.

I hereby declare my financial freedom NOW and henceforth forever!"

#BlastOffTips

Play the Warmer-Colder Game! Do you remember that childhood game called "You're Getting Warmer, You're Getting Colder?" That's where someone hides something, and then you search for it while being told, "You're getting warmer," "You're getting hot," and "You're burning up," as you near the object.

The more relaxed and playful you are the better. Feelings of abundance will give you a warm glow; feelings of lack will give you a cold shudder. Just remember you're getting colder and colder with negative emotions and pushing abundance further away.

The greatest power you can ever develop is the ability to focus on the abundance and good in your life right now; mastering this skill alone can make you one of the richest people on the planet!

9.

SELF TRANSFORMATIONAL TOOLS

I'm hugely passionate about sharing tools to enable and empower people to help themselves and my experience has taught me that simplicity is the key in self-help and personal development.

In my first book Love Life, Live Life I covered a whole chapter on Letting Go and in that explained how EFT Emotional Freedom Technique (also known as Tapping) had helped me.

In this chapter I am sharing more powerful (some may see as slightly random!) techniques that have worked so well for me and countless others.

Even if you feel some do not resonate with you right now or you feel you don't need to use any of them, trust me they are very powerful and worth referring to as and when required.

If, of course, you believe you need "outside" help, there is an abundance of amazing coaches, therapists and healers worldwide. Trust you will be drawn to the right one to assist you.

If you find yourself embroiled in anything that

triggers negative emotion, I always say to people "remember to use the tools!"

As I mentioned in Chapter 4 when you have an emotional reaction or trigger to someone or something you may think that you can't control your emotional reaction.

If you allow that emotional reaction, it's called a refractory period.

If you allow it to last for a few hours or days that's called a mood.

If you keep that same emotional reaction going on for weeks or months (for example, holding onto bitterness or negative emotion about something that happened months ago) that's called temperament.

Keeping that same emotional reaction going on for years on end is called a personality trait.

We now know the impact negative emotions can have on every area of our life and so learning how to shorten the refractory period of your emotional reactions is key.

Remember, if you feed the negative emotion it's like adding fuel to the fire and all you are doing is disempowering yourself.

Holding on to resentment, anger and bitterness is like drinking poison and expecting the other person to die!

Not feeding the emotion and letting it go does *not* mean you are condoning someone else's behaviour; you are empowering yourself.

Ho'oponopono - Hawaiian Healing Practice

Years back this Hawaiian healing practice didn't resonate with me at all, however since 2013 I've become a huge fan of this very simple, yet powerful healing tool.

It is a self transformational technique that can work miracles.

Ho'oponopono (meaning to "make right") is an ancestral Hawaiian practice that was used as a form of family therapy. This old Hawaiian practice was simplified and adapted by Mornah Simeona and has been popularized by people like Dr. Hew Len and Joe Vitale who featured in The Secret. The practice is so simple and so powerful that it is difficult to believe the results one can achieve.

Ho'oponopono can be learned in 5 minutes, implemented immediately and practiced anywhere, anytime. It's a simple form of mantra, affirmation or prayer (call it as you like) that doesn't require adopting a new belief system, it's not bound to any religion and encompasses love, responsibility, respect, forgiveness, faith and gratitude.

We are the sum total of all our experiences and when we experience stress or fear in our lives, if we were to look carefully, we would find that the cause is actually a memory. It is the emotions which are tied to these memories that affect us now.

What this process does, quite simply, is clean the data, which is stored subconsciously.

Mornah Simeona describes the main purpose of it is to discover the Divinity within oneself. She believes it is a profound gift which allows one to develop a working relationship with the Divinity within and as we do it our errors in thought, word, deed or action are cleansed.

It has proven so effective that she taught it at the United Nations, the World Health Organisation and institutions of healing throughout the world.

A big part of Ho'oponopono is about taking personal

responsibility and the understanding that "peace begins with me". The world is a reflection of what is happening inside us. If you are experiencing upset or imbalance, the place to look is inside yourself, not outside at the object you perceive as causing your problem. All that takes place in your life is created by your memories be it at a conscious, subconscious, cellular or soul level.

Every stress and imbalance can be corrected just by working on yourself. Ho'oponopono permits you to clear away your memories. Memories are not intrinsically bad or good; we make that judgement about them. It may be that the memory of an event seemed good for years (for example, a marriage) but we now remember it as bad (it ended in divorce).

Some memories appear to be false and others seem accurate. However, they are all only memories that need to be cleansed of the negative emotion so you can be free of them. Ho'oponopono makes this possible.

The Mantra and how this cleansing is performed.

"I love you, I'm sorry, please forgive me, thank you"

Some people choose to start with "I'm sorry" but I agree with Joe Vitale that when you start with "I love you", you are immediately connecting to your higher self and I find this to be more powerful.

You begin with "I love you", it immediately creates that connection to your higher self, only love can heal and when you say this you are speaking to both your memories and yourself.

Then you say "I'm sorry" because you were unaware that you carried that memory inside of yourself or sorry for your part to play in this (at some level).

Then you say "Please forgive me" to the divinity you carry within yourself and ask the divinity for assistance in self-forgiveness that you allowed these memories to "lead you astray".

Next you say "Thank you" to your memories for appearing to you and thus giving you the opportunity to free yourself of them. You also thank the divine and your inner divinity for helping you in this liberation.

This process is to forgive yourself, thank yourself and send yourself love. By doing this you erase the impact of the memory. As the suffering vanishes from within you, it also disappears from the other person or the situation. When you speak these words you are addressing yourself, specifically the young child within you who is in pain.

You have nothing to do or understand other than just to say these words.

Anytime you have a trigger of a negative emotion, gently repeat the mantra for as long as you feel is necessary.

This is particularly what I love about the simplicity of Ho'oponopono. It is no longer necessary to hunt for the source of a disruptive memory, the painful event surrounding its origin.

The process can seem difficult to the mind, only because the mind wants to control and understand everything. But your mind is useful in this process and plays an important role. The mind has its own free will and it can make the decision to let go of all control and power and place its trust in the inner divinity to clean out and therefore free you of your memories. The intellect mind gives way to the intuition of the heart.

The mind functions in the same way as a computer; it uses your past memories for data. The mind always refers back to them before making any decision, whether that's consciously or subconsciously, and as touched on in previous chapters ensures that you are living your life according to patterns dictated by the past.

I'm always reminding people to *not* judge their future results on their previous experiences and this is a great tool for assisting in this.

When you stop judging and using the recipes of the past, you will be living in the present moment and be prepared to welcome a new reality.

This new reality will no longer be under the control of your ego but under the guidance of your soul.

**To summarise; there are 2 ways to live your life....
from memory or from inspiration.**

Memories are old programmes replaying and inspiration is the Divine giving you a message. To hear the Divine it is important to "clean" the memories.

Do it on your own and you can say it thinking of anybody, anything, any situation, issues, self, your body, disease, illness, crisis, God, the Universe, humanity and so on.

I know people who have used this powerful mantra with family members in mind, a scenario that happened a long time ago that kept triggering the same response, creating upset or anger

They took 100% responsibility that the memory was stored within them and they cleaned it in the amazing Ho'oponopono way. In no time at all, the situation healed and they connected joyfully as a family without justifying, arguing or "micro" managing the situation.

As mentioned in Chapter 8 Manifesting Abundance, if your financial situation and/or your business is creating stress for you Ho'oponopono it!

It's powerful, trust me!

Tapping the Thymus Gland

Here's another quick self-transformational tool for your total well-being mind, body and soul; tapping the Thymus Gland. I recommend doing this daily as part of your getting up routine.

The Thymus Gland was named from the Greek word "thymus" which literally translates into "life energy". The Thymus is located in the middle of our chests, just above our breasts, you know when you've found the spot, it can feel slightly sensitive.

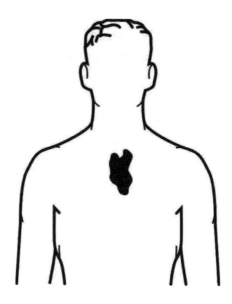

It is responsible for manufacturing and releasing T-cells which are an important component of our immune system. T-cells are involved in our overall wellness, helping our bodies to resist diseases like cancer.

The thymus is a major part of our immune system. In addition, the thymus also creates a connection between mind and body and is sensitive to emotion, stress and negativity.

When we experience high levels of stress, negativity and an imbalance of emotions we are more prone to illness. One thing we can do to increase health and wellbeing in our bodies, even in times of great stress, is to stimulate the thymus gland.

Tapping the thymus boosts energy, relieves stress and increases strength and vitality and is a part of many ancient healing traditions.

For a speedy burst of energy, tap your thymus with your fingertips for 20 seconds, while slowly and deeply breathing in and out.

Don't tap too hard. You only need gentle tapping to stimulate the thymus gland.

Some experts suggest that in order to have the most energising effect tap in the waltz beat, a one-two-three count, with the emphasis on the first count, repeating the affirmation "My life energy is high, I am full of love."

In addition to strengthening the immune response in your body, this technique can also be helpful in pain reduction and can be used as and when required.

As you tap you can say some of your own positive affirmations, for example, "I am healthy, mentally emotionally and physically" but I particularly wanted to share it with you in this chapter as it is a powerful way to release any fears and blocks that you may not be consciously aware of.

I was shown this by a very gifted spiritual teacher

and friend, Donna Maxine, and the mantra she taught me to use while tapping, which I did every morning as part of my daily routine, is as follows;-

"I now willingly and lovingly release any fears and blocks that I may have at a conscious and subconscious level, through all time and space that may be holding me back at this time, and I now willingly and lovingly step into my greatest, happiest and most abundant self" (or whatever positive words you may choose to use there that resonate with you).

Of course, as you say it, you can add fears and blocks around money, or fears and blocks around relationships or your health or whatever you feel is relevant to you in the moment.

It's our life energy and when our life energy is vibrant and strong, our awareness and our connection to source is enhanced too.

Breathing techniques for the mind, body and soul

One of my twin sons' Nick is a yoga teacher, amongst many things, and is hugely passionate about sharing powerful breathing techniques to aid total wellbeing; mentally, emotionally, physically and spiritually.

Thanks to Nick for this contribution.

"If you ever find yourself, for whatever reason, in a state of fear, worry, anxiety or depression where your mind is racing and perhaps you are going into overwhelm, try these breathing techniques. They are great wherever you are and you can do it without people noticing!

The incredible benefits to breathing are not commonly known. Out of all of the automatic functions of the body, only one can be easily controlled voluntarily – our breathing! This acts as a portal, a way into our nervous system and gives us the ability to gain some influence over how it performs.

Just to explain and keeping this simple without getting too "sciencey", within our entire nervous system there are two parts that play an important role in how we think, feel and function; the sympathetic (SNS) and parasympathetic (PNS).

The sympathetic gets you ready to do the things you need to do, as well as to respond to threats or danger by releasing adrenalin (our fight or flight response), speeding up the heart, increasing our breathing and getting us revved up and ready to go.

The parasympathetic is the counterbalancing part, which helps to slow down our heart rate and our breathing, calms the mind, restores energy and enables us to relax (our rest and digest, relaxation response).

We need both parts in our daily lives; at times we need more of one and less of the other. For the majority of our day, ideally, we should have a balance of the two.... enough get up and go (SNS) with a balance of the calming role (PNS).

Unfortunately with the busy lifestyles we all lead and so much potential distraction, we are finding that we are spending too much time in our revved up energising part of our nervous system, the SNS. This then leads to chronic stress, anxiety and not feeling so great.

Before the Coherent Breathing technique below, a great soothing and calming technique is the 4-4-6-2 breath counting exercise.

Simply breathe *in and out* through your *nose*, filling your lungs and closing your eyes if appropriate to do so. Inhale whilst silently counting to 4, you then hold for a count of 4, exhale for a count of 6 and then hold for a count of 2.

This is a full breath cycle; repeat this for 5-10 minutes if possible. This will calm you and help to reduce or stop a racing mind of negative thoughts from taking over.

If it's initially too uncomfortable for you to slow your breathing down all the way, then start at a pace more comfortable to you. In time your body will adjust with more ease and relaxation.

It is important though to keep to the specific ratio and breathing pattern as best you can, as this has significant impact on how well they work. The longer time on the exhale stimulates the relaxation response.

The following technique is known as Coherent Breathing, simply put it helps the main systems of the body, such as the nervous system, cardiovascular, respiratory, digestive, hormonal, glandular and immune systems align and work in harmony with each other.

Coherent Breathing

Part of what makes this breathing technique so effective and why I love it is its ability to increase the health of your Vagus Nerves.

Keeping things simple and brief this set of nerves make up the majority of your soothing and relaxation nerves (PNS). The vagus nerves, vagus meaning "wanderer" in Latin, come down from the brain stem, through our neck and split and wander all around your chest and abdominal cavities innovating virtually all our internal organs from our brain, areas of our neck and throat, lungs, heart, kidneys and all the way down to our gut.

These nerves play a vital role in our day to day functioning as a healthy human being, not just on a physical level but mentally and emotionally. They affect our overall well-being, from a healthy regulated heart beat and blood pressure, breathing, improving our digestion and immune system to relieving depression and anxiety. They manage the release of oxytocin; the hormone responsible for bonding, connection and compassion.

We all should want healthy vagus nerves also known as a high vagal tone. High vagal tone = a happier healthier you... low vagal tone = a not so happy or healthy you!

There are multiple ways to stimulate and increase the health of these healing nerves and the following technique is rather easy and straightforward to do.

The Technique

1. Bring your awareness to your breathing and if appropriate to do so close your eyes and relax your arms.

2. Focus on the subtle sensations of the air passing in and out through your nose and into your lungs. If your mind begins to wander no problem just bring your awareness back to the sensations of your breath.

   Breathing should be gentle and relaxed.

3. Begin to slow your breathing down.

   It's important to remember to breathe **in and out through your nose**. If for any reason breathing through your nose creates difficulties, breathe through your mouth with "pursed" lips, i.e. gently touching with a small gap.

*** As the nose is a smaller air passage way in comparison to the mouth, it has a natural calming and slowing effect on the breath. It also helps clean and filter the air and regulate carbon dioxide and nitric oxide, two gases that have a vital role in healthy and happy breathing, the benefits of which are greatly reduced with mouth breathing.

Yes, there are times when breathing through your mouth might be the only option, for example, sinus problems, a blocked up nose (or when running or exercising hard).

There are also some effective breathing techniques where you exhale through the mouth, but for general day to day life try to breathe in and out through your nose as there are so many more overall benefits.

For the breathing techniques I'm sharing with you here ideally for maximum benefit keep or switch to nasal breathing as soon as you are comfortable to do so.

4. As you take conscious control of your breathing rate, aim to extend your in breath and out breath to a count of 5 to 6 seconds each. Do this gradually so that you remain comfortable.

In the beginning if 5/6 seconds feels too long and uncomfortable, reduce to a comfortable count and increase with practise.

***Breathing at this rate is known to maximise heart rate variability (HRV) and the electrical rhythms of the heart, lungs and brain become synchronised. The greater your heart rate variability, the more balanced and toned your nervous system is, resulting in a happier and healthier you!

5. As you inhale it's vital to use your diaphragm and the easiest way to do this is to take your breath down into your abdomen so that your belly and ribs expand.

    TIP: Initially in the beginning I suggest to gently place one hand on your belly and the other on your upper chest as you breathe. Your hands act as markers to see and feel what parts of your body you are breathing with.

5. As you inhale your belly will expand, followed by your ribs and a slight lift in your chest. At the top of the inhale, without pausing, gently start to exhale. Your chest will soften, followed by your ribs and then your belly. This is known as one complete breath cycle.

    ***Notice if you are holding any unwanted tension in your body, in your shoulders, neck, your jaw and muscles in your face. If you find any tense areas, consciously take a full in breath, contract the area, followed by a prolonged exhale and physical release and letting go. Continue the body scan and the feeling tends to dissipate.

Breath Moving

You may find that when doing the coherent breathing your mind and thoughts may tend to wander. If so why not incorporate into this practise what is known as breath moving. This will help to increase focus and improve concentration of the practise.

1. Very simply as you breathe in imagine you are moving your breath up to the crown of your head.

2. As you breathe out imagine your breath now moving down to the base of your spine.

3. Each time you breathe in move your breath to the crown of your head.

4. Each time you breathe out move your breath down to the base of your spine.

Breathing in this slow controlled way, as if you were in a place of safety and comfort, sends signals to the brain that all is well and helps restore balance at every level of your being.

The longer you can continue to breathe at this rate, the greater the effects. Even just a few minutes can do the trick.

Think of this breathing technique not only as a coping mechanism in times of stress, but also as a daily practice and exercise. It will truly build a mind and body that can adapt and adjust to any challenge that may come your way and sustain inner calm and peace.

Most people notice benefits immediately. You will notice that your mind feels calmer, less filled with chatter; your body feels more relaxed. In the beginning, these good feelings may last only a short time after you get up and start doing things under the usual pressures. However, with practice over time, the benefits will last longer and longer the sense of calm alertness will grow, and the feelings of tension will fade.

This wonderful technique can be used any time of the day, but for maximum benefit I would suggest you do it as part of your morning routine to prime yourself for the day ahead and again in the evening.

Of course, if you are at all concerned about any

health issues you may have, please consult your doctor beforehand.

Nick Stone

Huge thanks to Nick for sharing one of his incredibly beneficial techniques. It took me a long time to really understand and "get" just how effective "right" breathing can be.

Meditation

The huge benefits of meditation are well documented and as I explained in Chapter 4, countless studies confirm that the practice of meditation permanently strengthens the most evolved portion of the human brain, the frontal lobe. This is linked to increased abstract thought, cognitive reasoning, creativity and positivity.

It also triggers the brain to release naturally occurring neurotransmitters, including dopamine, serotonin, oxytocin and endorphins, which are linked to different aspects of happiness from simple pleasure to a deep sense of calm.

Regardless of your religious orientation or which method you choose to meditate, sitting still for even five minutes a day can help you clear the mind, confront and minimise negative conscious and unconscious thinking patterns and connect to the divine space within that transcends thoughts, feeling and circumstance.

Through practice meditation will enable you to experience the stillness of the field of pure limitless potentiality; the ultimate ground of creation where everything is inseparably connected with everything else.

There are many different ways to meditate, so if you haven't found one that feels right for you, keep looking!

Some of the more commonly known methods include transcendental meditation, prayer, Zen meditation, Taoist, mindfulness, walking meditation and Buddhist meditation. Several of these require your body to remain still, while others allow free movement.

I find I "tune" in very well when I'm out in nature, walking and totally present in the moment. I simply focus on the natural abundance surrounding me, the blue (or cloudy) sky, the trees, I listen to the birds and I imagine with every breath I am taking in pure positive source energy into my system.

Some people find it easier to meditate and get in the "zone" with music, either with gentle movement or being still.

Listening to the Dalai Lama, he explained that meditation is something within us; it's a state of being that we learn. Eventually we can learn it so well that we *become* it 24 hours a day. We want to condition our minds to live in the present moment, not in the past or the future.

He made me understand that meditation doesn't need to be a strict practice, either; you don't have to have an altar filled with gifts; you don't have to sit erect on the floor or in a chair; if you have an itch, by all means scratch it! Our culture wasn't meant to practice the way monks do, nor does meditation need to have a religious connotation.

Give yourself permission to let go of expectation, and understand that meditation doesn't have to take more than five minutes of your day. If you can manage *one* minute, that's an accomplishment and it's something to build on. You may just find that you thrive on the all round benefits so much that you meditate for 30 minutes twice a day!

Start by closing your eyes and taking four deep, long breaths, on both the inhale and exhale and then breathe normally. When your mind jumps around, wanders or starts chatting excitedly about anything, breathe out, mentally tell it "later," and let yourself return to the quiet.

Or follow Dr. Joe Dispenza's technique I cover in Chapter 4. Talk to your body as if it was a dog you were training. If you can sit your body down and tell it to stay like an animal, stay right here, I'm going to feed you when we're done or then you can get up and check your emails and texts etc but right now you're going to sit here and obey me!

I find just focusing on my breathe helps keep me in the present moment. You can also use a mantra or phrase that you mentally repeat in your mind slowly, putting as much focus on that as possible, even as you do it casually, almost relaxed.

Don't judge your performance or allow yourself to get frustrated. Don't get discouraged either. This is not a contest. Very few people on the planet can get their minds quiet for a whole minute or two!

Over time, this practice will become easier and more natural. You will enhance your intuition, raise your energetic vibration and contribute to a happier, more uplifted experience of yourself, others and the world at large.

Five Steps to Access Your Heart's Intuitive Wisdom

One of the things I've been focusing on over the years is to develop my intuition. I've learnt to trust my gut feel and "nudges" and the key is to then act on this inspiration.

Just as it is possible to turn on our televisions and radios and tune in to a channel of our choice, we also can create coherence between our brains and hearts and trigger the deepest possible states of intuition when we choose.

It's our ability to trigger our deep intuition consciously and intentionally that awakens the wisdom of the heart.

The following exercise is one of those places where science and spirituality overlap beautifully. While science can describe the close relationship between the heart and the brain, the ancient spiritual practices and self-mastery techniques that have helped people rely on this relationship for thousands of years do so without needing a scientific explanation.

It's probably no coincidence that the rigorous scientific techniques developed by the researchers at the Institute of HeartMath closely parallel some of the techniques preserved in the monasteries of ancient traditions or by indigenous spiritual practitioners.

With this in mind, I've chosen to share the following IHM technique (www.heartmath.com), with permission, because it's safe, it's based on well-researched science that validates the steps, and it has been simplified in a way that makes it accessible and easy to use in our everyday lives.

Step 1: Create Heart Focus

Action: Allow your awareness to move from your mind to the area of your heart.

Result: This sends a signal to your heart that a shift has taken place: You are no longer engaged in the world around you and are now becoming aware of the world within you.

Step 2: Slow Your Breathing

Action: Begin to breathe a little more slowly than usual. Take approximately five to six seconds to inhale, and use the same pace as you exhale.

Result: This simple step sends a signal to your body that you are safe and in a place that supports your process. Deep, slow breathing has long been known to stimulate the relaxation response of the nervous system (aka the parasympathetic response).

Step 3: Feel a Rejuvenating Feeling

Action: To the best of your ability, feel a genuine sense of care, appreciation, gratitude, or compassion for anything or anyone. The key to success here is that your feeling be as sincere and heartfelt as possible.

Result: The quality of this feeling fine-tunes and optimizes the coherence between your heart and your brain. While everyone is capable of evoking a feeling for this step, it's one of those processes that you may need to experiment with to find what works best for you.

At this point, the heart and brain are in communication through the neural network that connects them.

It's from a state of heart-brain coherence that we may access our deep intuition and receive the guidance of our heart's intelligence.

Steps 4 and 5 below detail a procedure to do that.

Step 4: Ask Your Heart a Question

Action: The previous three steps create the harmony between your brain and your heart that enables you to tap into your heart's intelligence. As you continue to breathe and hold the focus in your heart, it is time to ask your question.

Heart intelligence generally works best when the questions are brief and to the point. Remember, your heart doesn't need a preface or the history of a situation before the question. Ask your question silently, as a single and concise sentence, and then allow your heart to respond in a way that works for you.

Result: Your intuition opens up and you begin a dialogue.

Step 5: Listen for an Answer

Action: Become aware of how your body feels immediately as you are asking your question in step 4. Make a note of any sensations- such as warmth, tingling, or ringing of the ears- and emotions that may arise. For people who are already attuned to their bodies and their hearts' intelligence, this step is the easiest part of the process. For those who may have had less experience in listening to their bodies, this is an exercise in awareness.

Result: Everyone learns and experiences uniquely. There is no correct or incorrect way of receiving your heart's wisdom. The key here is to know what works best for you.

Even if you don't get an answer straight away, that's fine too. Just relax, trust the process and be open to receive the intuitive "nudge" or knowing in due course. As with many things, practice makes perfect!

Don't forget this quote I mentioned in Chapter 6, which many attribute to Albert Einstein. "The intuitive mind is a sacred gift and the rational mind is a faithful servant. We have created a society that honours the servant and has forgotten the gift".

Slowing your brainwaves down and tapping into your intuition enables you to work "smart" not hard. I love this analogy which explains this well.

Alpha Brain Wave benefits

If you imagined you had a super duper sports car, you wouldn't just get in it, put it in first gear, and put your foot to the floor and race around all day, would you? If you did that what would happen? The engine would eventually burn out!

This is exactly what most people do on a day to day

basis, racing around, constantly in the alert state known as beta brain wave. This is exactly the same as having your foot to the floor in first gear. What this will eventually do is burn our systems out. We all know what stress is. When we are stressed our immune system shuts down, we become ill, lose focus and it's a downhill spiral.

We know that in the car If we were to change into second gear, the engine would quieten down but the wheels would gain momentum. You go into third gear and fourth gear the same thing happens; the engine quietens and the wheels gain momentum.

I cannot stress enough the importance of finding this time to relax, to calm and still your mind and body. You in turn then are in flow, more intuitively guided and gain momentum in life without the old paradigm of pushing and forcing things to happen.

Sing

Singing is a natural anti-depressant (whatever your singing sounds like) and is known to release endorphins, the feel-good brain chemical that makes you feel uplifted and happy. Not only that, but singing can simply take your mind off the day's challenges to boost your mood.

Singing also releases stored muscle tension and decreases the levels of the stress hormone called cortisol in your blood stream.

When singing, improved blood circulation and an oxygenated blood stream allow more oxygen to reach the brain; this improves mental alertness, concentration, and memory.

Get creative

Creative activities relieve stress, aid communication and help arrest cognitive decline.

The beneficial effects of creating aren't dependent on a person's skill or talents. It's the process, not the product, so get creating or join a class. There's so much out there on offer covering such a wide range of activities.

#BLASTOFFTIPS

When you are challenged, feel stressed or trigger any form of negative emotion, remember to use the tools!

10.
NOT GETTING YOUR DESIRED RESULTS?

Over many years I've connected with tens of thousands of people who are aware or becoming aware of the power of their thoughts, emotions and beliefs; the ancient wisdom backed up by science, which has also become known as the Law of Attraction in relatively recent times.

Despite their best endeavours, it's become very clear to me why people do not get their desired results. It can vary between some "fine tuning" to a complete overhaul. I'm a straight talker and very passionate about helping others. My intention in writing this chapter and covering this issue from lots of angles (and overlaps) is purely to help the reader, to help you, achieve your desired results.

There's no point knowing what to do; you must do what you know

It's all very well reading books, going on programmes and courses and knowing the theory, but if you don't actually practice it and apply it into your daily life *consistently*, you are just not going to get the results.

167

I love Gregg Braden's take on this and it purely reaffirms my belief that this "stuff" *must* become a way of living if you truly wish to see real change in your life.

"When we talk about the practice for many people in the West it sounds like something that we do "sometimes". The key to all of the traditions is that it becomes a way of life rather than something that we do sometimes.

Our conditioning in the West is that our "spiritual" practice is something that we do at the end of the day, when the children are fed, the bills are paid, the dishes are done, the clothes are clean and the lunches are prepared for the next day. Then we go into a room, close the door and turn on the music, light the incense and burn a candle and by then it's two o'clock in the morning and we're too tired to do anything.... we take a deep breath and say a mantra and go to bed!

That's an exaggeration, but for many people the point is that their spiritual practice is compressed into a few moments after everything else is finished in our culture, ours being the West.

However, you go into the Native American cultures in North America, South America and into the monasteries in Egypt and Tibet, their entire lives are the spiritual practice. It's just the opposite of the way we think about life.

So again it's about becoming the practice and allowing it to be a way of life rather than viewing it as something that we do in a moment in time. We do programs all over the world and people come, soon after the program they say "Great program, when is the next one? What should I study next?"

I have to say to them there is no more. Go home and experience and live what it is that you've learned here. But for some people the diversion is easier to go from workshop to workshop, study to study and teacher to teacher rather than embrace and live what they've learned already in their lives"

Daily Disciplines for A Positive Way of Living

Here's a summary of my Daily Disciplines to incorporate into your positive way of living.

1. As you wake up in the morning and are in the sleepy state of Alpha Brain wave (when the door is open to the subconscious mind) spend five minutes getting into the "zone" of gratitude and love; a wonderful vibration to start the day on.

Set the intention "Today everywhere I go I create a peaceful, joyful and loving world"

2. Once you are up, calmly and with positive intention tap on your thymus gland repeating the following powerful statement, as explained in more detail in Chapter 9.

"I now willingly and lovingly release any fears and blocks that I may have at a conscious and subconscious level, through all time and space that may be holding me back at this time, and I now willingly and lovingly step into my...* greatest, happiest and most abundant self" (*or whatever positive words you may choose to insert that resonate with you).

3. Through the day be consciously aware of the thoughts that you are thinking and the statements you are making.

Identify any negative and self-limiting thoughts and beliefs that you are having. Be kind to yourself. Don't "feed" them; convert your inner critic to be your inner coach and replace them with powerful positive affirmations (more suggestions below) and encouraging self talk of "I CAN do this!"

4. Utilise healing/letting go techniques and self transformation tools through the day as appropriate and when required.

I've included some hugely powerful ones in Chapter

9 that can help you at a conscious, subconscious and soul level.

Too many people forget to use the tools when they are experiencing any of the negative emotion spectrums. They purely end up feeding the negative and fuelling the fire. This in turn stops you healing and moving forward in life and blocks or repels your desired results.

You have the power to self heal and reprogramme yourself! Believe it!

5. As I have covered throughout this book, find some time daily to relax and nurture yourself. Meditate and still your mind; BE in the moment.

There's no such thing as a bad meditation, there's only overcoming yourself!

6. Be aware of your thoughts and visualisations last thing at night as you fall asleep. This is a hugely powerful time.

Make this the *last* thing you do before you fall asleep. Gently inhale to the count of 4 and exhale to the count of 4, repeat until you feel relaxed or alternatively find some calming music on YouTube or similar to listen to.

Visualise and think about positive things only, don't beat yourself up going back over your day and what you perceived as not going right!

Give your attention to one particular thing you wish to manifest. See yourself in your mind having already achieved the outcome and hold this vision for at least a couple of minutes.

If you find it challenging to visualise, relax and thank the universe, thank God and/or your angels for bringing this desire into your reality. Also give thanks for the good in your life *right now*.

This is alpha state and a powerful time to fall asleep calmly and gently repeating to yourself your key "feeling" words – happy, calm, healthy, free, love, abundant, prosperous, confident, successful etc.

This is particularly useful if you have had a "challenging" day. Just pick out the single word that is relevant to what you feel you need in the moment. As you gently and calmly repeat it you are "drip feeding" the seeds in your subconscious mind. What you sow you reap.

When I was going through my dreadful and fearful period around money I would quietly repeat in my head "wealth, abundance, wealth, abundance" and so on.

Whatever you do, don't go and watch the TV, a video or listen to the news after this process as this may well be in opposite alignment to what you are trying to manifest!

A shortcut to creating the life you love!

The "shortcut" is to nourish your mind with *powerful positive feeling* words of how you would feel once you have achieved your goal. This gives new instructions to your subconscious mind and the universal intelligence. With practice you start to feel these elevated emotions in the now.

Remember, this is ancient wisdom backed up by science. The heart is the strongest biological generator of electrical and magnetic waves and is 5,000 times more powerful than the brain magnetically!

Dare to dream! Open yourself up and tap into the pure limitless potentiality.

What would it *feel* like once you have created a life you love?

What would it *feel* like once you are in a wonderful

loving relationship?

What would it *feel* like once you are enjoying vibrant health?

What would it *feel* like once you have your dream job?

What would it *feel* like once you are running your own business?

What would it *feel* like when you have just delivered a fantastic speech and received huge applause?

What would it *feel* like once you are truly making a difference in the world?

What would it *feel* like once you have financial freedom?

What would it *feel* like once you are living in your dream home?

What would it *feel* like once you....(fill in your own goal)?

Make a note of the "feeling" words that come up for you; a very beneficial exercise.

Write out your "life mission statement" (sample

below) incorporating these words (providing they are positive, of course, which I would like to think they are!).

Dare to dream that you could actually create a life you love and live in that vibration consistently; effortlessly gliding through any of life's challenges that may come your way....with, perhaps, the perfectly acceptable occasional "wobble" or "human moment" as I would call it.

This IS possible, believe it!

(Please don't misunderstand me here, by "life's challenges" I'm not, of course, referring to any bereavement, loss of loved ones and world tragedies or similar).

Switch your mentality from the negative self talk and embrace some of the following statements that are appropriate for you in any moment, especially if you don't feel you're ready to fully embrace the powerful "life mission" statement, below, just yet.

Always say them in the positive and present tense "I am" not "I will be" ("will" is always in the future!).

"I am not broke and miserable anymore" does *not* work. The subconscious can't tell the difference between the negative and the positive; it will merely take "broke and miserable" as your instructions.

Whatever negative word you have been using, flip it over to the polar opposite. It may feel strange to begin with but that's ok. Remember the meadow analogy.

Your mind's job is to do what it thinks you want and it bases that on the words you use and the pictures you put in your head.

Starting with *every day in every way and in every moment* is a gentle but progressive introduction to the subconscious mind, depending on where you are now and how you are feeling.

Every day in every way and in every moment I love and accept myself more and more and I am enough.

Every day in every way and in every moment I am growing and healing.

Every day in every way and in every moment I am open to feeling more positive and happy. I am grateful for all the good in my life right now.

Every day in every way and in every moment I am finding it easier to be more and more positive.

Every day in every way and in every moment I am creating the life of my dreams knowing that I am supported by the universe at all times.

When you feel ready, embrace and go for this longer one below, or tweak it to suit with positive language that resonates with you. You can also repeat "bite size" sections from it as appropriate throughout your day.

Example of a "Life Mission" Statement

Every day in every way and in every moment I am so grateful for all the amazing good in my life right now.
I am totally happy and I am at peace.
I am whole, right here right now.
I am confident, empowered and fulfilled and I am abundant and successful in all areas of my life.
I am thriving and I am free. I am love.
I am vibrant, energised and healthy, mentally, emotionally and physically.
My life is flowing better than I ever imagined possible.
I love life and life loves me back!
Thank you, thank you, thank you!

A thought and statement repeated over and over again eventually gets accepted as a belief.

As I've already shared, my personal favourite at the

time of writing this book is...

I am rich beyond my wildest dreams, I am, I am I am
I am rich beyond my wildest dreams in love and joy and
health and wealth.
Thank you, thank you, thank you!

I believe and feel it all to be true and it's exactly what has manifested in my life. By adding "beyond my wildest dreams" is allowing my manifestations to evolve and expand without limits.

As soon as you can, introduce some super duper power words such as passionate, thrilled, ecstatic, phenomenal, awesome, amazing, fabulous, thrilled and so on. Elevate and amplify the e-motion.... energy in motion!

By *deliberately choosing* positive grateful and loving thoughts you create positive grateful and loving feelings. Your feelings in every moment are what you are creating for your future..... more things to love and be grateful for! (*Quantum Physics*).

Every time you deliberately change your thinking you are growing new neurons. See it as a seed bed and as you say things baby neurons start to grow just like a green shoot. Each day, create your day and say repeatedly the same positive things. Expand

and add to it all and these little shoots start to grow (*Neuro Science*).

These little shoots (baby neurons) grow and contain the sentence/affirmation you are saying and as they grow they move and connect with the consciousness of that potentiality.

Research demonstrates that it can take from just a few days to 42 days to create new neural pathways and if you keep at it you become hardwired; what you say is what you are and the reality you are in!

You have to be able to do it enough that you neurochemically, through repetition, condition your body to understand the feeling (that you're working towards) as well as your conscious mind does.

If you keep doing it *over and over and over and over and over again* (and the more elevated emotion you can feel as you are speaking, the better) you'll activate the part of your brain called the cerebellum, the seat of your subconscious mind; the home of your habits and your skills.

Remember to allow yourself a transitional period as you shift your consciousness and raise your vibration.

Your shifts and changes can be very subtle sometimes. You may have a situation that you suddenly become aware how differently you have responded to it. "Wow only a few weeks ago I got so anxious/angry and now it's happened again I've dealt with it in such a different way without even thinking about it!"

Most people can't be bothered to put the "work" in or don't understand the importance of the repetition, a major reason for not getting their desired results.

However, we know that if we want to be good at anything we have to practice and train. If you wish to be good at tennis, for example, you can buy the most expensive racquet, some top designer trainers, a lovely frilly skirt or shorts and watch some videos and read many books. However, if you don't get out on the court and keep practising, you know you will never get really good at it!

It's the same with training our mind to think positively.

I love the analogy of learning to drive a car. Here in the UK (and in other countries) we can't drive alone until we have passed a theory and practical test. When we start learning to drive we have to think about every little thing, every step of the way.

We might stall, get in a fluster, argue with the person teaching us, we may even bump the car as we are learning and get totally frustrated! However, more often than not we don't give up! We keep practising and practising because we *know* and can *see* the tangible freedom it gives us when we pass our test.

Freedom is the word here! If only people realised the freedom we create when we release ourselves from the "chains" of our old limiting and negative thinking and beliefs.

It's the most amazing feeling! I truly had forgotten what it felt like to be happy years ago. At the time of all my dramas and crises I could never have dreamt of the life I now enjoy and feel very blessed that I have done so consistently over many, many years.

Of course, as with driving a car, once the behaviour becomes learnt the subconscious mind takes over and we don't have to consciously remember to indicate or look in the mirror, we do it automatically. Likewise I don't have to "work" at being positive anymore, it's automatic.

So please, please don't give up. I promise you it's worth it! Obviously we are thinking tens of thousands of thoughts a day, hence why living consciously throughout the day with a moment by moment awareness, where possible, is the key to faster tangible results.

Practice, practice, practice; repetition, repetition repetition. If I can do it, trust me, so can you!

The way you FEEL in EVERY moment is what you are creating for your future!

This is definitely a key phrase to remember and forgetting or being unaware of this is a major reason why people do not achieve successful and rewarding manifestations.

They may do their affirmations, their visualisations and meditations etc in the morning or late at night and the rest of the day get "caught up" in the drama, stress and frustrations of the day. The predominant energy they are radiating throughout the day is stress and frustration; this of course creates more things to stress about and be frustrated with!

If you spend half your day positive and half your day negative, it's a bit like mixing acid with alkaline; it totally neutralises the whole situation with no overall change.

If your thoughts are chaotic and all over the place consider the instructions you are sending out into the universe and your subconscious mind.

Identify your limiting beliefs

Many people do not get their desired results because they have not identified their limiting beliefs that are holding them back.

I've reiterated throughout this book that a "moment by moment" awareness (as best you can throughout the day) of what you are thinking, feeling and saying is key to identifying any subconscious self-limiting and negative beliefs that have been holding you back.

Once you are aware of them, you are half way there!

If you *believe* your problems are too big to solve, you will not "see" the solution.

If you *believe* this is your "lot", it will be.

If you *believe* you are "stuck" or "blocked", you will be.

If you *believe* you can heal yourself, you can.

If you *believe* that to be successful in your business or career your personal life will suffer, it will.

I could go on and on with many different examples here but I cannot stress enough the importance of identifying those beliefs. They indeed may well have been born out of good meaning and intentions, but you do not have to take them on as your "truth" anymore.

Write it, say it, see it, feel it

If you haven't already, get yourself a journal or special note book. The following process will definitely boost your reprogramming and the successful manifestation of your desires.

Allow yourself some "me" time, relax and if possible light a candle.

In your book, each day, write down your "inner you" feeling affirmation/life mission statement (as above in the present tense as if you have already achieved it) and any other physical or material goals you have.

Do the following;

Head the page up "Day 1".

Do this whole 3 step process one statement/goal at a time.

1. Write your first statement/goal down. As you write it, notice the words individually as they are created. When you are writing you are using the left hemisphere of your brain and thinking in "words".

2. Put your pen down and declare your statement out loud with positive emotion; sound propelled with positive emotion is a hugely powerful vibration in the universe.

3. Visualise and see yourself in your imagination having already achieved your goal and living the life of your dreams; remember, you are the director of the movie of your life, in your mind, so please direct a movie you like the ending of!

See yourself loving life, in full colour and play this movie/vision in your imagination. When you are visualising you are using the right hemisphere of your brain and thinking in "pictures".

The key when visualising is to really get into the emotion of how amazing you are going to *feel* once you have achieved it. This aligns your vibration beautifully for success. This may take a bit of practice but keep practising! Passion is a key ingredient for success.

It's important to hold the vision and emotion for at least a couple of minutes, this then becomes strong enough for a vibrational match in the universe.

The more you can feel these positive emotions throughout your day, the more consistently you are in a vibration of allowing and receiving; a "win win" all round for your mind, body and soul.

The interesting part here is that you have a band that connects the left and right hemispheres of your brain, called the Corpus Callosum. When you use both hemispheres of the brain in this way, this band becomes like a super fast broadband service. The information and inspiration "download" is so much quicker!

Repeat the 3 step process on your next goal if you have more than one. I don't recommend having too many goals to write down, as you don't want this process to become a chore if it takes too long. Anywhere from 1 to 5 is easily manageable.

The following day head up the next page in your book "Day 2" and do exactly the same all over again; the same goals individually and the same 3 step process.

Continue for 42 days without a break. If you miss a

day, begin again at Day 1.... all part of effective re-programming.

(Don't forget to verbally repeat with positive emotion your affirmations and goals throughout the day... the more you do it, the quicker you create new neural pathways!).

Congruency

Every relationship in your life contributes to the overall vibration you are radiating. This includes all the different ways you relate to that which you desire, as an example, let's take money.

If you don't like your job and it doesn't pay you very well, and you try to manifest more money or another job, that probably won't work so well because each time you go to work at your job, you risk re-triggering the vibration of feeling financially under-appreciated.

This of course sends out conflicting vibrations every day for many people. They may visualise having more money and feeling abundant and grateful, but then they go to the supermarket, and they buy cheap, low quality food because in the back of their mind, they're saying to themselves that they can't afford the good stuff. That naturally cancels out the vibration of abundance, so the result is no change.

If your current circumstances cause you to emit conflicting vibes, then even as you go through the motions of acting in accordance with a scarcer financial situation than you would like, keep your vibration focused on that of abundance.

The best way to do that is by feeling the emotion and heartset of gratitude. So even if you buy cheap, low-quality food, hold the vibe that you're grateful for it and that you appreciate it. Feel appreciative that such food exists and that it's within your budget, and then look at the high quality food and emotionally invite it into your life.

If possible, find one way in which you can splurge for higher quality items, like buying a few organic apples or vegetables, and feel grateful that you can do that. When you eat those apples or vegetables, really enjoy them and set the intention to receive more of the same.

But please do NOT beat yourself up for not being able to afford what you desire. That will only lower your vibration.

Desire and detachment

From a personal point of view this is an area that I had to really work on. I had a huge desire for a particular outcome but I kept reading and learning that I must *not* be attached to the outcome! It totally confused me years back. Hopefully the following will give you some clarity if this is something you have been struggling to get your head around.

What is the relationship between desire and detachment? Aren't they diametrically opposed? How can you have both at the same time? Isn't desire a form of attachment?

No, these aren't in conflict. They co-exist perfectly. Let me explain.

Desire is about what you wish to create. You could describe this vibration as passion and excitement. It's an amazing sense of emotions you summon by focusing on a new vision and goal. The stronger your desire the better, so amp it up!

Detachment, on the other hand, is about *how* those desires ultimately manifest for you. When you become too attached to when and how your desires show up, you are not in flow and slow down or block the manifesting process. Instead of holding the

189

vibration of playfulness, excitement and abundance, you start sending out signals such as concern, worry, frustration and stress. Don't do that!

When you notice that you're getting frustrated, pause, breathe and go back to the desire side. Hold that vision of the creation you wish to experience, and indulge in the positive sensations of being there in your heart, mind and soul. Trust and know that physical reality will soon catch up, as long as you keep holding the right vibration. Feel the sense of gratitude as if it has already happened!

Vision plus *inspired* action is the key to manifestation

Forced action and trying to make things happen ends up creating a load of hard work and no positive outcome.

Inspired action is the action that you take when you feel inspired to do it. It's "in-spirit", intuitive action. These are the actions that you take whole-heartedly, with great enthusiasm, with good feeling and excitement and you feel a sense of joy in them. That's the receiving mode. You are in the zone!

When you feel moved and inspired to take action from a place of passion and excitement, not stress, then go ahead and let those actions flow through you. Follow your impulses. There may be some twists and turns and course re-directions along the way and that's fine and it's still progress!

Trust and believe, allow and surrender

This is a biggie for many and it certainly was for me in the beginning. I had zero trust in anything and no awareness of the power of this "stuff"! Once I got on the case and started "working" on myself and my thinking, one of my very first affirmations and positive self talk was "*I trust in the power and the magic of the universe*" and "*I believe in miracles, miracles happen to me*". I mention these in my first book Love Life, Live Life. I repeated and repeated them throughout the day and after a short while I began to believe what I was telling myself.

As I started shifting my thinking and visualisations to what I *did* want in my life rather than what I was fearing and what I didn't want, I became solution conscious as opposed to problem conscious. That's when "seemingly impossible miracles" happened, the right people were coming into my life at just the right time, money came into my life from unexpected sources and my trust and belief started building. I like to describe it in my experience as compound interest; started small and built on itself.

191

Where I see people not getting their desired results is when they have a great vision of what they would like to achieve, they know what to do, they visualise it, feel it and take some action towards it. BUT they spend more time thinking about and planning what they will do if they don't achieve their goal. Unfortunately, we get what we plan for!

Don't visualise success and plan for failure! Hold your vision and trust.

The key to all this is *not* to worry about the "how". That's what we trust the beautiful divine intelligent universe for. Remember, we are all connected.

As soon as you start to worry about *how* you will achieve your goal and over analyse it, you lower your vibration and potentially block your path to success. Most of us have been brought up to figure it out for ourselves, however that's the old outdated paradigm, and now we are aware of so much more.

I love this analogy which explains it well.

These days if we are driving somewhere and we don't know how to get there, what do we do? We get the post code or zip code of our destination and promptly put it into our sat nav on our phones or in our cars.

We then relax (allow and surrender) and totally *trust* that the intelligence of the GPS will calculate the best route for us to take.

We don't worry and go into overwhelm about what we are going to do nearer to our destination (generally anyway). We happily (hopefully!) get into our car, turn on the engine, put it into gear and gently put our foot on the accelerator. Lots of small necessary action steps.

Too many people go into overwhelm worrying about how they are going to achieve their goal and end up not going anywhere fast.

All you can ever do in the Now is take lots of small inspired action steps in the direction of your goal. *Relax* and *trust*, *believing* that the macro intelligence will guide you intuitively and show you the way. As I've previously mentioned it can be hard for us humans to trust in something we can't tangibly see, however we trust the air we breathe and we can't see that (well unless it's freezing cold of course!).

In your car you may come across a road block. In that moment you have a choice; give up and go home or sit quietly and allow the intelligence of the GPS and a bit of common sense to show you the best course re-direction.

Even if it may take you longer to get there, remember to enjoy the journey! THIS moment right NOW is all you have got, so choose to embrace it positively.

Setting "big" goals

So many people say to me they are successful at asking the angels for a parking space and manifesting small goals, but they can't manifest "big" goals.

If we see goals as "big" at some level we believe they are out of our reach and we are not worthy. We are therefore not vibrationally aligned and it cannot come into our physical experience. Treat this contrast as inspiration to improve.

The same thing applies if we spend too much time focusing on the "lack of" something and the "not" having it now.

Give yourself permission to deserve and expect a great outcome no matter what.

Do the vibrational work first. *Feel* the version of you that has everything you desire.

If it feels way off, see it as if you are trying to turn a

juggernaut around. Lots of tiny tweaks and manoeuvres get you there!

The joy is in the journey. The manifestation of any goals is just the start of a new journey. Focus on the fullness of now and be satisfied and grateful, i.e. in a state of allowance and trust in the unfolding of it.

My Timing versus Divine Timing

Divine timing is something that can be a huge challenge for even the most faithful and trusting person. No matter what you are trying to manifest, you can't escape divine timing (I tried!).

It can be annoying, especially if you are urgent about your manifestation. Divine timing is a lesson in patience. There are several things that go into this. First of all when you are feeling the urgency about having something, you are sending out the energy of desperation, which will block the manifestation immediately.

However, this doesn't mean it is blocked forever. It's only blocked as long as you are desperate or urgent about getting what you want. The universe has a plan for you. The universe knows us way better than we know ourselves. It knows our divine life purpose, it knows what is aligned with your life purpose and it knows what would be the very best thing for us.

The universe wants us to have a happy, successful, prosperous, purposeful and fulfilling life. The universe wants you to have your heart's desire. The big difference between you and the universe is that the universe has the bigger view and knows the bigger picture, while your view or picture of reality is limited to your experiences, knowledge and belief system, i.e. what is in your consciousness. Of course the ego loves to kick in everywhere it can too!

When you are starting to get impatient and no longer want to wait for the universe to make its magic, or if you think your plan is better than the universe's, then it is your ego that takes the lead. When your ego takes the lead you are ruled by fear based thoughts and emotions. These lead to fear based actions that very often take you on a detour instead of speeding up the process.

Your manifestation should be aligned with your life purpose. We all have a life purpose, some big, some small, some involving our personal development, some involving making a difference in the world. The universe will never give you something that would not serve your life purpose or support your current learning.

Life is about learning and developing and every day brings new opportunities to grow. Sometimes what we are trying to manifest is not the right fit at this moment in time. We're just not ready for it, even though we think we are! It would be like sending a child in nursery school or kindergarten to the exam in sixth form or high school and expecting the child to pass with high grades.

You must count free will into the equation.

You cannot interfere with the free will of anyone or anything. You can't force things to happen if everyone involved does not agree upon the outcome, whether that is consciously or unconsciously. If you do try to force something to happen, even if the universe doesn't give you the resources you need and the people involved don't agree upon it, there may well be some interesting repercussions.

Your own free will also plays a role. It's great to want something, but you must be willing to take the appropriate action to receive it.

So one of the reasons you have not got what you want right now is because you haven't made the necessary changes to align yourself vibrationally with your desired outcome. Instead of getting frustrated and impatient, spend the time working on yourself and raising your vibration.

Ask for signs

Impatience often comes from not seeing any proof of manifestation. Getting frustrated if you can't see any signs is like stamping on the corn as it hasn't popped up yet!

At any moment you can ask the Universe or God to send you a sign, something like this message I say.

"Dear Universe, God, Angels, my guides..... (or whatever and whoever feels right for you, I'm not going to make a judgement or decision on that).

Please and thank you in advance for sending and giving me signs in this physical world that are easy for me to notice, recognise and understand and that shows me the manifestation is on its way to me. If there is anything I should know or do please nudge me and make it obvious and clear to me so that I can take the right inspired action. Thank you, thank you, thank you!"

Then relax, surrender and let it go! The universe knows exactly which signs to send you and is more than happy to do so. Be patient and allow yourself to be surprised and grateful by their creativity.

Let go and hand it over to the universe.

You must get out of your own way. Every time you are trying to control the outcome you actually say to the universe that your plan is better than the divine plan. Because of your free will the universe hands you the wheel and puts you in charge. Are you ready for that? Are you ready to figure out everything on your own and accept the delay in your manifestation that it causes? Let go of control and your life will change.

Our intelligent universe already knows what to do and the moment you hand it your desired outcome, it starts to work behind the scenes. The universe can activate other people, circumstances, opportunities and situations to help you fulfil your heart's desire. Control is a resource that you don't have nor should you try to have it because that could be manipulation.

If you're trying to manifest a romantic relationship, for example, with the perfect life partner, you have to take into consideration that the other person also has free will and also needs to be ready to be with you and be a good partner for you. Those things can't be forced.

The universe knows when everyone involved, for

the greater good of all, is ready for the manifestation to happen. So hand it over to the universe, surrender and let go and follow the divine guidance you receive every day and trust on the perfect outcome at the perfect time for all concerned.

Forgetting to plug yourself in?

I love these analogies from Abraham and Esther Hicks about the importance of gratitude and reaching for the thought that feels best in this moment right now. Gratitude is the power cord to the universe. Don't forget to plug in to get the best results!

"When you take action before you've done anything about hooking up with the universe, it would be like deciding that you're going to toast some bread for breakfast and you put the bread in but you don't plug the toaster in. The bread just sits there.... and you wait and wait and wait and wait and the bread never gets toasted because it's not plugged in!"

"If you get your vacuum out and don't plug it in, you create lots of marks on the carpet, exhaust yourself but you don't achieve your desired results"

The emotional signature of gratitude means you're getting something. If I give you something that's of value, you would say thank you because you would feel it. So, when you're receiving you're giving thanks, so gratitude is the ultimate state of receiving.

When you raise your vibration, there are about 1,200 different chemical reactions that go on in the body that begin to restore and repair the body in a state of gratitude. The research has been done to prove it.

It's a "win win" at every level; mind, body and soul!

#BLASTOFFTIPS

Don't see this as "hard work", have fun with it and be playful "Bye bye negative thought, you're not for me anymore!"

Tapping on the karate chop of your hand as you say your goals, affirmations and powerful positive self talk, helps embed them more quickly at a cellular level.

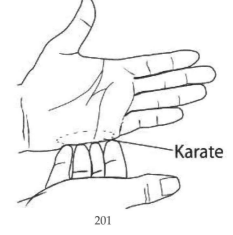

201

If life isn't flowing as you would like it to right now, work on your inner world and shift your vibration.

All positive emotional states including gratitude, joy, love or excitement means your state of being is one of allowance and receiving.

All negative emotional states including worry, frustration, jealousy or guilt means your state of being is one of resistance and blocking.

This book contains all the knowledge necessary to create a life you love. If knowledge is power, the knowledge about yourself is self empowerment. The *application* of this knowledge is key to attaining your desired results and in no time it will become an effortless way of living and loving life!

Simply see your subconscious mind as a Ferrari and your conscious mind as you, the driver. Once you learn how to, you can handle the Ferrari with ease. See yourself as a highly skilled and competent Ferrari driver.

Master yourself and you master your life!

11.
Rocket Fuel for Your Body – Living Younger Longer

Did you know that positive thinking can actually make you live longer?

Research has found that people who have a positive attitude and embrace aging, rather than dread growing old, have a greater chance of living longer. That's because adjusting your perception of aging, especially while you're still young, improves your positive outlook and can have a tremendous effect on your life expectancy.

Researchers believe that positive thinking about aging can increase a person's will to live, making him or her more resilient to illness and more proactive about health and well-being.

Most of us are no stranger to health problems, illness, or pain but wish we were. And most of us would love a new lease of life with the ability to live disease-free, have more energy and enjoy greater well-being.

Is that possible, though? Is it too late to even try? Yes, it *is* possible, no it's not too late but it's not just looking for answers in the conventional medical environment either.

The answers are within your own body. Your body has a built-in capacity to heal itself; a remarkable system of self-repair that goes on day in and day out. Improving its ability to heal is within your control.

Health comes from the *inside* out and not from the *outside* in.

Think well, feel well, be well

Love, laughter, joy, hope and any number of positive emotions are hugely healing, by contrast negative emotions, such as worry and anger do just the opposite; they block the healing energies of the body.

Every thought you think is heard by every cell in your body

That's a statement worth remembering! This is one of the reasons why so many people have chronic health problems. How often do we hear people continually talk about what's wrong in or with their bodies?

I've already shared the scientific experiment in Chapter 3 about a gentleman in a B29 bomber in

World War 2 and how his cells reacted years later; it's worth remembering that every cell in your body responds perfectly to every thought and emotion that you have. Positively or negatively!

Lifestyle and attitude is key

If you haven't already come across Bruce H. Lipton, PhD I recommend you take a good look at his work. He is an internationally recognised leader in bridging science and spirit, a stem cell biologist and bestselling author of The Biology of Belief amongst other great books. This is what he has to say.....

"It's a scientific fact that less than 1% of disease is connected to genetics. Over 90% of cardio-vascular disease is lifestyle and attitude. Diabetes type 2 is an epidemic which is nothing to do with anything wrong with the body; it's all lifestyle and attitude. It's all down to your programming and belief. It's the negative people that get in the way of creating a positive world. Ignore the negatives and do your own positive work and then you can create miracles and your own heaven on earth."

The relationship between emotions and healing is not just a mind game or a matter of semantics. There is a true physical relationship between your emotions and nervous system, endocrine system and immune system. What you feel turns into the chemistry, biology and the immunity of your body.

So much of what goes on in your body is under the control of peptides and receptors. When you feel happy, your brain produces happy peptides; when you're sad, your brain produces sad peptides.

Peptides travel to cells and enter them through doorway-like receptors. Once inside, they influence many of the cells actions. For example, they might cause your face to turn "white as a sheet" when you are scared or "beetroot red" when you're embarrassed or enraged. They do so by regulating blood flow and signalling receptors on blood-vessel walls to constrict or dilate.

Every hour of every day millions of cell divisions occur in your body to replace the old cells that die. If someone feels sad for just one hour, they have produced billions of new cells that are more sensitive to depression-type peptides. Those new cells are creating a body that is more apt to feel depression than joy.

Since your body is remaking itself like this all the time, doesn't it make sense that you'd want to produce more happy peptides than sad ones? Of course you do! You can do this by creating the best possible emotional health you can. Love and gratitude are powerful and it might be as simple as just smiling or laughing more.

Those positive thoughts transform positive emotions, producing happier peptides, which will visit your cells and keep your body in a state of emotional equilibrium.

There's power in a hug too! Hugs are self-healing. Science has verified that the simple act of reaching out and hugging another person slows heart rate, reduces blood pressure and even accelerates recovery from an illness. All that in a simple hug!

Through my research I've come across so many powerful stories of common people all over the world in all different cultures doing the uncommon. They're healing themselves from disease, including chronic and potential fatal diseases.

This one story below is truly powerful and gives hope and inspiration to many. Thanks to Dr. Joe Dispenza for sharing it.

"This particular lady had experienced a very sudden loss, a trauma. This in turn produced very strong emotions which lingered for a long period of time. It's a scientific fact that the hormones of stress push the genetic buttons and create disease, and the long-term effect of living by

those chemicals are harmful to our bodies.

In a very short amount of time she developed paralysis from the waist down, which in turn created more stress in her life. She couldn't work, she couldn't take care of her children, she couldn't make any money and she couldn't take care of her house. She had to get assistance from other people and her mother had to move in with her.

Stress on top of stress she developed ulcers, she could no longer eat properly and within three to four months she developed Oesophageal cancer.

This woman was smart enough to realize that probably the effect of those chemicals were the reason why she had developed her condition.

She said to herself if I created this condition because I was living by this event, emotionally attached to my past, is it possible then to uncreate it and create something else.

So she began the "work" during meditations every single day, whether she felt like it or not. For sure she had certain days where she didn't feel like doing her meditations, even when she didn't feel well she did them anyway. She also made the decision that she wasn't going to stop her meditations until she was in love with life.

Now to the materialist, who defines reality with their

senses, there's no reason for her to be in love with life for obvious reasons. But she said I'm going to teach my body emotionally what my future could feel like before it's made manifest.

Every single day she overcame a small part of herself and within a very short period of time, about a year, she was able to reverse all her conditions.

To this day this woman has none of the symptoms, she has a new life! Her new personality created a new personal reality. The disease exists in the old personality.

If you talk to this woman about that experience she'll tell you that the experience was her greatest teacher."

Wow, what a powerful true story, an amazing lady and true inspiration, don't you think?

It's wonderful to know that positive thinking and positive emotions create powerful rocket fuel for your body to enable you to live younger and healthier for longer, but what else can you do to help yourself?

The benefits of improving fitness and how to do it

I asked a great friend and valued member of the Sue Stone Foundation, Denise Sargent, to contribute her amazing knowledge and experience on fitness.

Denise is a Personal Fitness Trainer; her specialist areas include cardiac rehab, diabetes, obesity and pulmonary care. She has run several full marathons, loves long distance cycling and, to stretch herself, she decided in her 50's to compete in Bikini and Fitness competitions, very successfully and has amassed an array of medals and cups!

Thanks to Denise for this contribution

"Rocket fuelling your body for fitness is one of the best things you can do for yourself. You could be completely starting from scratch or improving the fitness you already have. Exercise can slow down, stop or even reverse the decline in the cellular health of muscles that comes with ageing.

We all know we should exercise but lots of people find it's easier to make excuses. The gym is expensive, boring, or a bit scary and intimidating. There's not enough time or I have too much to do, I don't enjoy it the list goes on.....

Looking after you however is far more important than any excuse. Getting fit doesn't have to be expensive.

So just for a moment, imagine being in great shape, imagine having an amazing amount of energy and getting the most out of every day, every moment. Imagine looking the best you have done in years. Imagine getting a real buzz out of life.

For so many of us these things seem impossible, something we used to have when we were young.

What happened?

We live in an amazing body; its every desire is to keep us alive and feeling great. It is an incredible design. But it seems we have forgotten to read the owner's manual. If you bought a beautiful new car and put dirt in the fuel tank, ran out of oil and never had a service it would soon feel like an old banger!

Well that's exactly what we do to our bodies, and then we wonder why we feel like old bangers, haha!

Let's add some rocket fuel!

Hydrate

Drink plenty of water. Water is critical for healthy bodies; it regulates body temperature, keeps joints mobile maintains youthful looking skin and aids digestion. Often we can confuse hunger for thirst, most people who are obese are dehydrated. So drink plenty of water to improve health and reduce weight. Try to drink two to three litres of water a day.

Exercise

Exercise improves your health and happiness and is vital for total wellbeing; mentally, emotionally and physically...... the list of benefits is seemingly endless:-

A great natural antidepressant

Reduces the risk of disease

Keeps your joints supple

Lowers the risk of Diabetes

Lowers the risk of Alzheimer's

Reduces high blood pressure

Aids digestion

Improves balance and coordination

Increases metabolism

Reduces visceral fat; the dangerous fat around the organs.

Reduces cholesterol

Builds healthy bones

Improves posture, suppleness, flexibility, balance and coordination

Maintains your lymphatic system

Strengthens ligaments and tendons

It extends your life

Walk in the fresh air

Getting out in to daylight even when it is not sunny will increase vitamin D absorption and make you feel more energized. Vitamin D helps regulate the amount of calcium and phosphate in the body. These nutrients are needed to keep bones, teeth and muscles healthy.

Walking is a great way to exercise and release mood boosting endorphins. Get out into the outdoors and get some fresh air into your lungs.

It's easy to get started as you don't need any special

equipment. Just commit to walking every day, or at least five days a week for 20 minutes, leave your front door and walk for 10 minutes then turn around and walk back.

If you work you can do this in your lunch break. Everyone can make 20 minutes for themselves, even if it means setting the alarm clock earlier.

If that's too much for you to start with, then walk five minutes out then five back. Whatever you start with increase it by two minutes per week until you are up to thirty minutes per day.

Remember day by day inch by inch and it becomes a cinch!

If that's too easy for you try power walking, start off with five minutes normal walking and then pick up the pace for fifteen to twenty minutes then finish with five minutes back at a normal pace.

A suitable pace to burn calories is three and a half miles an hour. To increase this try an incline walk.

Always wear comfortable clothes and flexible shoes. Swing your arms, bent at the elbow so work your upper body. You can think of your arms as pumps when you go uphill.

As you walk calm your mind, become aware of your breathing and slow it down. Relax your shoulders and look straight ahead.

Be thankful for being alive and reflect on things that make you happy. When I walk I look up to the sky and thank the universe I'm alive, sometimes I shout this out loud but only when I'm in the forest, not on the high street!!

I immerse myself in the sensations of nature, listening to bird song, or smells of fresh rain washed earth. My favorite smell is cut grass, it's odd how a smell can make you happy but it does.

If you have the opportunity, again not on the high street, try barefoot walking. Walking on sand and grass feels so lovely but also you can absorb electrons from the earth through the soles of your feet. This practice is called grounding or earthing.

This technique can help with sleep and pain relief and also strengthen muscles because we walk as nature intended.

Try new thinking; think about feeling young and energetic. Don't let negative thoughts hold you back; thinking differently about yourself is the way to make real changes in your life.

Try new things

Try new things and find out what you enjoy doing; dancing, walking, cycling, swimming or an exercise class could be the change you need.

Find a challenge to motivate you if walking is not enough try something else. Find something you actually look forward to doing or makes you feel fantastic afterwards.

All areas now have park runs (see www.parkrun.com for information on this all over the world). They are held on Saturday mornings in local parks here in the UK and are free. The distance is 5km and you register online. They give you a timed finish and so you can challenge yourself to improve.

Yoga is a great way of relieving aches and pains and reducing stress. If you don't feel ready to join a class you must at least stretch. Watch your pets or animals, when they wake they stretch.

You can even do a few stretches while you are boiling the kettle for your morning cuppa, it doesn't have to take long and you will feel the benefits.

Increase your grey matter

Neurologists at Stanford medical school studied brain scans and found that people who exercised regularly had increased grey matter in the prefrontal cortex which governs stress management.

The grey matter includes regions of the brain involved in muscle control and sensory perception such as seeing and hearing, memory, emotions, speech, decision making and self-control.

So start or keep that exercise going! It's also clinically proven to stimulate the positive endorphin serotonin. This lifts your mood and enables you to cope with stress. Serotonin is your natural feel good neurotransmitter.

Remember when embarking on any new regime do not "see" it as "hard" work or that you are depriving yourself.

Deliberately focus on the benefits, affirm and visualise yourself vibrant, energised, healthy and happy!

Remember the quote made famous by the late Dr. Wayne Dyer, "When you change the way you look at things, the things you look at change" (This is quantum physics!).

"Be excited to rocket fuel your body with
exercise, positive energy and great nutrition"
- Denise Sargent

The power of plant-based nutrition

One of my twin sons' Rich is a plant-based wellness advocate. He is passionate to the core about sharing his knowledge of the true power behind plants and how this diet and lifestyle can ultimately have such a positive impact on your life and the lives around you.

Thanks to Rich for this contribution

"I have been fascinated by the power of plant-based nutrition and how it has been successfully used for decades in the treatment of chronic disease and general health and wellbeing.

I have been studying the work of some of the true pioneers in this space, such as Dr Neal Barnard and his success with reversing Type 2 Diabetes, Dr Caldwell Esselstyn with preventing and reversing Coronary Heart Disease, as well as a number of other key figures successfully treating auto immune issues and even certain cancers through plant-based nutrition alone.

Diet is powerful stuff and can have dramatic results in both positive and negatives ways.

I am extremely excited to share with you some of the knowledge that I have collected over the years that I believe are essential to living a more healthy and fulfilled life!

The current health situation in today's society

First let's briefly touch on the current health situation that we face today and look at what's really going on!

In today's society we are literally plagued with chronic disease, just look around you; Cancer now affects one in two people. Heart Disease being our leading killer and Type 2 diabetes is rapidly affecting most of western civilisation. Not to mention the increasing number of auto-immune issues we are seeing more and more of these days.

This is not normal! Something has gone seriously wrong with the way we live our lives and human health today as we know it. If you stop still for just a moment and take a look around you, how we eat and live our lives has changed so much over recent years. Humans eating habits have changed more in the past 50 years than they have done in the past

10,000.

We no longer eat the fresh produce from our garden and local farms, but instead we consume highly refined and processed foods that our bodies just do not know what to do with.

Just look at all the refined carbohydrates and processed fats we run through our bodies, not to mention our high animal product in take. The majority of us now consume animal based products at every meal, not even our Palaeolithic ancestors ate animal products three times a day.

No wonder our cholesterol and weight has gone through the roof. Cholesterol is only present in animal products and saturated fat tends to only be found in them in high amounts too.

Our bodies actually manufacture both of these naturally, the problem occurs when we consume them in higher amounts through our diet.

Our desire for meat and all animal products in general has led to severe environmental consequences, including habitat destruction, species extinction and now has even led to ocean dead zones where all forms of life now ceases to exist. Not forgetting that if you took one look at the majority of farms today and saw how these animals are kept and treated it would probably make you think twice about your food choices.

So what is a plant-based diet anyway?

A plant-based diet is a diet based on foods derived from plants, including legumes, whole grains, fruits, vegetables, nuts and seeds, with few or no animal products.

Let's start with the main food groups that we base our meals around, these include legumes (all the different types of beans, peas and lentils) whole grains (such as quinoa, buck wheat, bulgar wheat, rice and oats) fruits, vegetables, nuts and seeds.

Not forgetting some of the beautiful tasting herbs and spices from around the world that you can include in any type of dish and cuisine that you can think of; Indian, Thai, Lebanese, Mexican, French you name it! Over the past few years of eating this way I have truly enjoyed experiencing all these amazing global dishes that are packed full of vitality and life.

One huge benefit of eating this way is that we get all the essential nutrients that our body needs for optimal health without the high levels of saturated fat and cholesterol found in animal products.

The aim here is to eat these foods in their "whole" form, just how it was grown. When we focus on eating whole foods we are eating the whole plant in its natural form which includes all the fibre and its nutrients that our bodies know how to work with.

Fibre is so important, not only is it essential for healthy digestion and for regulating our body to absorb nutrients, it also plays a major role in removing potential carcinogens (a substance capable of causing cancer in living tissue) from our food as well as excess cholesterol, hormones and fat that may be circulating in our body.

The amazing benefits of incorporating more plant-based foods into your diet is the powerful medicinal properties that are naturally found in plants; just some of these include immune boosting, detoxifying, anti-inflammatory and even anti-cancer effects.

The side effects of eating a plant-based diet

Your blood pressure and cholesterol begin to drop, that extra weight around your waist starts to melt away, and your insulin sensitivity improves! Not to mention the increase in energy you will experience from all those natural colourful plant foods now in your diet.

Apart from the high amounts of nutrients present, plants contain water and fibre which is so powerful at assisting healthy weight loss. All you have to do is eat until you're full, there is no calorie counting.

That is the power of fibre! You see fibre fills you up way before you ever get the opportunity to over eat and consume those excess calories.

Key nutrients essential for great health

Let me briefly explain a couple of key differences about fats. Saturated fat tends to be solid at body temperature which is primarily found in all animal products. I for one certainly don't like the idea of solid fat particles running through my blood vessels clogging me up. Just think about that for a moment!

That, along with cholesterol, are the two main culprits that cause atherosclerosis, a disease in which the inside of our blood vessels become damaged and narrow due to the build up of plaque. Like I mentioned earlier, our bodies manufacture their own saturated fat, the problem starts to occur when we consume too much of it in our diet.

We should be more focussed on consuming healthy

unsaturated Omega 3 fats in the form of Flax and Chia seeds, dark leafy greens, legumes and whole grains. These are essential to good health; our bodies cannot make them and must be consumed through our diet. Omega 3 fats are liquid at body temperature which allows them to glide effortlessly through our body.

Common confusion around carbohydrates

I also want to briefly touch on carbohydrates; there is some serious confusion when it comes to carbs. I hear all too much these days that "carbs make you fat!" Or that "carbs are evil!"

Let me explain, when we consume a carbohydrate it is digested and broken down into glucose (sugar) which our body uses for energy. Our bodies love glucose; it is the preferred energy source for human beings.

Our organs, muscles and even our brain loves glucose. If we have very little amounts of glucose available our bodies will even convert protein into glucose it is that essential to our health!

The issues lie when we cast one big net over the entire carbohydrate family. You see, table sugar is a carb, white bread is a carb, cakes, biscuits and lots of other snack foods are also carbs!

However so is a beetroot, sweet potato and so are blueberries, bananas and apples! They all technically fall under one family however there is a huge difference between the first group and the second.

The first group which includes table sugar and snacks consist of highly refined and processed carbs that are unnatural and wreak havoc on our bodies and drives inflammation.

We experience spikes in our blood sugar which then result in sudden crashes in energy. All the essential nutrients and fibre have been stripped away during the processing resulting in a concentrated toxic form of sugar.

We want to do our very best to eliminate these types of foods from our diet, your body will thank you!

Now the second group however which includes sweet potato, berries and bananas are absolute nutritional powerhouses just how Mother Nature intended us to eat them.

They are loaded with antioxidants which protect us against oxidative stress brought on by diet and lifestyle. They also have alkalising and anti-inflammatory effects on the body. They are what we call a "whole food"; perfectly intact and full of essential nutrients and fibre which aids healthy digestion and absorption. These types of foods are truly power foods for our bodies and should be included in our diet on a daily basis.

So next time you read that carbs are bad; you'll be able to make a more educated and hopefully healthier food choice.

Protein sources on a plant based diet

In case you are concerned about where you would get your protein from on a plant-based diet, like I originally was, let me quickly explain a couple things and put your mind at rest.

There is so much protein present in plants that if you eat a varied plant-based diet you will consume more than enough protein for optimal health.

Animals don't make protein; they simply consume it through their diet.

Plants actually make protein; they do so via a function known as photosynthesis. The only reason why a steak has protein in it is because the cow that was once grazing in a field, ate the grass that contained protein which then was digested and stored in the muscle of the animal. It's not until you eat the steak that you then take on and store the protein that originated from plants!

For anyone who leads an active lifestyle and may require higher amounts of protein, then your go to foods on a plant-based diet are the legume family. These guys are absolutely loaded full of protein, even your dark leafy greens, nuts and seeds contain healthy amounts of protein.

Misconceptions around Vitamin B12

Finally I want to touch on something I get asked quite frequently when people enquire about eating a plant-based diet and that is Vitamin B12.

Vitamin B12 is essential to good health. It supports the nervous system, red blood cells, your energy levels and more. B12 is a bacteria found throughout nature, it's in our soils, rivers and streams.

One big misconception is that people believe you have to consume animal products to get B12. As with protein, animals don't actually make B12, they get it through eating vegetation and drinking from the streams.

Back in the day humans naturally got lots of B12 in their diet through the water they collected and the soil particles found on fruits and vegetables.

However due to today's over farming, which has led to the soils being depleted of B12 and our sanitation procedures, our water supply and fresh produce is now cleaned, which in turn kills off all bacteria including B12.

This is not a big deal as you can get healthy sources through fortified foods and supplements, such as B12 liquid drops you put under your tongue and/or in pill form. I personally use the drops as they are more easily absorbed.

A little bit on iron

Iron is an essential mineral, it is a type of metal just like zinc and copper that we need to live and survive. These essential minerals come from the earth and soil. Plants absorb them through their roots and store them in the plant itself. Humans and animals alike then eat the plants and store the iron and other metals in their bodies, which can then be used for a number of bodily functions.

Iron plays a major role in red blood cell production and in the transferring of oxygen from our lungs to our muscle tissues throughout our body, as well as other great things.

As stated iron is essential, however there is a strong body of evidence within the medical and scientific communities, showing a link between too much of these metals in our diet and the potential damage that can be caused to our brain and body health.

Let me explain, iron, like copper, is an unstable metal; pour a little water on one of these soft metals and watch the colour change. This is known as oxidation, similar to when you cut an apple in half and leave one half of it on the side exposed to the elements. It begins to darken.

Another example that always comes to mind is as children we would throw pennies into water fountains and make a wish. Did you ever notice why a lot of the pennies already in the water fountain had turned dark and rusty?

This also can happen inside our bodies too, yes we need these essential minerals to survive, however, too much of them can have adverse effects.

If we have too much iron in our bloodstream this can wreak havoc and cause oxidation. Oxidation is the production of free radicals, which are highly destructive and unstable oxygen molecules. They can damage our brains cells and accelerate the ageing process, just like the darkened apple and the rusty pennies.

There are two types of iron; non-heme and heme. Let's take a quick look to understand some key differences between the two and which one is overall healthier for us as human beings.

Iron is present in pretty much all plants, in particular dark leafy greens, legumes, sesame seeds, pumpkin seeds, quinoa and dried apricots. This form is non-heme iron.

If we happen to have plenty of iron in our blood already, our body is able to turn down its absorption of the non heme iron from the vegetables we eat, and if we're running low our body naturally pulls more of the vegetables' iron into our bloodstream.

Heme iron is found in our meat, particularly beef, pork and lamb. Animals get iron from the grass they eat which then becomes concentrated in their blood cells and muscle tissue.

It is much harder for our bodies to regulate heme iron, even if we have more than enough iron in our body already.

If we aim to reduce our meat intake and increase our fruit and vegetable intake, we will get all the iron we need without the potential health risks.

A powerful health tool

Let's now touch on something that I find truly fascinating about different foods and which is another key component to optimal health.

A powerful health tool to know and understand is the acid versus alkaline foods. Knowing this can really help transform the way you look at food and make food choices! What most of us aren't taught about nutrition and human health is that certain foods have an alkalising effect on our bodies and certain other foods have acidic effects.

Our bodies run optimally in an alkaline state, preferably ph 7.3 give or take. What we are sadly not taught is that animal products, meat, fish, dairy and eggs and refined carbohydrates, including alcohol and the table sugar, snacks and cakes I mentioned previously, are very acidic and create inflammation in our bodies. This in turn creates the "perfect" environment for chronic disease to set in.

However, the majority of all plant foods like your dark leafy greens, fruits and vegetables have amazing alkalising effects on our bodies. The more colourful plant foods that we include in our diet will lead to the benefit of a more alkaline state. This in turn keeps our bodies healthier and stronger to help protect us from illness and disease.

Eat the colours of the rainbow

Aim to eat the colours of the rainbow. That doesn't mean you have to eat 10 different colours every day but at least throughout the week try to mix up the colours on your plate, in your bowl or smoothie /juice.

Every colour has a unique and powerful healing property that does the body the world of good. For example, the orange coloured pigment that is present in carrots and sweet potato helps support our immune system and is also a powerful antioxidant.

The dark green colour found in spinach, kale and other greens helps our bodies to build healthy new cells and genetic material. Whereas the blue and purple colours found in berries and grapes helps to protect us from free radical damage and even aid the body's natural ability to hunt down and destroy cancer cells.

There is no limit to what you can do when it comes

to a plant-based diet. So who would have thought that something as simple as what's on the end of your fork could be so powerful and life changing for you, the planet and the animals.

Recommended reading

www.nutritionfacts.org
www.pcrm.org
How Not To Die by Dr. Michael Greger, MD
Dr. Neal Barnard's Programme For Reversing Diabetes
Power Foods For The Brain by Dr. Neal Barnard, MD
Prevent And Reverse Heart Disease by Dr. Caldwell Esselstyn, MD
The China Study by T. Colin Campbell, PhD
Chris Beat Cancer by Chris Wark

"I wish you all the best and most of all enjoy the process!" Rich Stone

Recipes for vitality

My daughter Natalie is passionate about creating delicious whole food plant based dishes. I've asked her to share some of her tasty recipes (breakfast, lunch and dinner) for you to enjoy and boost your health, perk up your energy, raise your vibration and feel lighter.

Thanks to Natalie for this contribution

Good morning booster juice

Benefits - This is an overall powerhouse of a juice. All these amazing ingredients help to support and promote a healthy immune system, boost our body's natural detoxing abilities by removing toxins. This juice also can also help support healthier blood vessels and improve blood flow circulation.

You also get a wonderful hit of antioxidants from all those amazing colours which reduce inflammation and oxidative stress caused by diet, lifestyle and general everyday living. Not to mention the amazing cancer fighting properties that are in their too.

(2 days supply)
1 bag carrots
3 lemons
Large piece of ginger
2 turmeric roots
2 apples
2 whole raw beetroot
2 vine tomatoes
½ whole cucumber
2 celery sticks

¼ fresh chopped pineapple

Wash, prep and chop produce as necessary
Add produce to juicer one at a time
Stir well before drinking

Golden milk

Benefits Golden milk is an ancient Eastern tradition; it has been used in Ayurvedic medicine for centuries. The key ingredient is turmeric, a yellow spice popular in Asian cuisine which gives curry its yellow colour. The list of health benefits seems to be endless, it is mostly known for its anti-inflammatory effects which can help all types of joint pain such as arthritis due to its strong antioxidant properties.

This amazing drink can also support your immune system which helps to fight and protect your body from cancer, improve gut health and digestion. Not forgetting it has also been shown to support healthy blood sugar levels too.

(2 weeks supply)
100grams Ceylon cinnamon
100grams turmeric
1 teaspoon black pepper

2 tablespoons of coconut oil

In a pan, put the turmeric, cinnamon, the ground black pepper and half pint of water (for now). Bubble it all over a low heat stirring occasionally for about 15 minutes until it forms a sloppy paste, you may need to add more water to get that consistency.

Let the paste start to cool and then stir in the coconut oil.

Once cooled, pop into a jam jar or kilner jar, pop in the fridge and it will set. I use a large teaspoon every night in warm koko milk and the same every morning or mix in your superfood porridge for breakfast.

Superfood Porridge

Benefits A bowl of Porridge is such a great way to start your day! Not only does it provide a long lasting supply of energy, but oats have been proven to have powerful cholesterol lowering effects and can even help the body recover from certain cancers by removing excess hormones from our body.

The fibre present in porridge will leave you feeling fuller for longer and can help reduce the risks of naughty junk food cravings.

Incorporating blueberries and flaxseeds will help fire up the brain with healthy Omega 3 fats while supplying the body with a nice hit of antioxidants which can help fight free radical damage and prevent cancer.

By opting for a plant-based milk instead of dairy milk you instantly eliminate cholesterol and dramatically reduce the bad saturated fat from your diet, a far healthier way to go.

Choice of oats
Choice of plant based milk
Handful of blueberries
1 banana chopped
1 teaspoon golden paste (optional)
Sprinkle of flaxseed & linseed

Make your porridge as directed and then stir in the rest of the ingredients and enjoy.

Tasty Tomato Tostada

Benefits This Tostada will give you a nice hit of taste, colour and leave you feeling full and satisfied. It's also a great way to get some healthy fats from the avocado, antioxidants from the tomatoes and lemon juice in your diet. Not to mention the powerful cancer fighting properties from the red onion, garlic and coriander.

1 soft tortilla wrap
140g fresh sundried tomatoes diced
¼ red onion diced
1 avocado
Juice of ½ lemon
Small bunch of mint and coriander chopped
Salt and pepper
Vegan sour cream and Violife cheese (optional)
Fresh diced chilli
Handful of watercress

In a bowl mix the onion, tomatoes, mint and coriander. Mash the avocado until desired consistency; add the lemon juice, salt and pepper to taste and mix.

Pop the tortilla into a hot oven for 5 minutes to slightly warm. Once out, grate the Violife cheese onto it then sprinkle the tomato and onion mix all over leaving a space in the middle for the avocado.

I like to add my avocado mix to the middle and also sprinkle fresh chilli and then a few drops of the sour cream. You can either fold in half or eat open like a pizza with the watercress on the side.

Tabbouleh (gluten free)

Benefits This is a great way to get some healthy whole grains into your diet which play a key role in good health. Quinoa (which is technically a seed, however classed as a grain) was a staple in the Egyptian diet and is a well known source of good health.

It is loaded full of micro nutrients and is also a great choice of healthy carbohydrates, protein and fibre that will leave you feeling fuller and nourished for longer.

300g quinoa rinsed
2 vegetable stock pots mixed in 900ml boiling water
1 pack radishes thinly sliced
1 pack pomegranate seeds (between 200-300g depending on shop)
150g dried cranberries
3 sprigs of fresh mint chopped

Large handful of fresh parsley chopped
Large handful of fresh coriander chopped
Juice of 2 lemons

Add the quinoa to the bubbling stock water. Leave to bubble for about 30 seconds then lower the heat, add a tea towel fully across the top of your pot and replace the lid. Let it slowly cook, stirring occasionally. Around 12 to 15 minutes it should have absorbed the water and be fluffy and soft. Add the sliced radishes, pomegranate seeds, dried cranberries, chopped fresh mint, parsley and coriander and then squeeze 2 whole lemon juices over it and mix well.

Sweet Potato and Quinoa curry- medium spice

Benefits Not only is this dish full of flavour and colour but it will help fuel your body with the goodness that it needs. This dish also has an abundance of nutrients that can help support your immune system, lower cholesterol, balance your blood sugars and fire up your metabolism.

(Serves 4/6 as a side dish or 2 as a main)
300grams of quinoa – rinsed
600ml water

1 veg stock pot
1 red onion – diced
2 sweet potatoes – peeled and diced
250g frozen peas
2 teaspoons of garam masala
2 teaspoons of cayenne pepper
2 teaspoons of madras curry powder
2 teaspoons of cumin
2 tins chopped tomatoes
Salt and pepper to taste
1 teaspoon fresh garlic
Bunch fresh coriander
Sprig of mint
Alpro soya yoghurt (plain)
¼ whole cucumber grated

Peel and dice the sweet potato and lightly season with some extra garlic granules, cumin and cayenne and roast for 15 minutes or until soft.

In a pan fry the onions until slightly soft on a medium heat, add the quinoa, the veg stock pot, the water, all the spices, peas and the tinned tomatoes.

Gently bubble away on a low heat stirring frequently. You may need to add a touch more water depending on the cooking speed of the quinoa.

It takes about 20 minutes for the quinoa to cook with

these extra ingredients to become light and fluffy but may need slightly longer. Mix in the cooked sweet potato, salt and pepper to season.

Sprinkle the coriander on top of the curry to taste. Mix the grated cucumber, yoghurt and chopped mint into a bowl for the cucumber raita and serve on the side.

Lentil Bolognese

Benefits This lentil bolognese is a great healthy alternative to the traditional minced meat version. By choosing a plant-based option you eliminate cholesterol and greatly reduced the bad saturated fat in your diet.

This heart healthy dish is loaded full of protein and a great source of carbohydrates that can help keep you leaner and full of energy, while helping to lower cholesterol and blood pressure.

(serves 4)
1 brown onion, diced
2 cloves of crushed garlic
2 large carrots, finely sliced
2 celery sticks, sliced

200g chestnut mushrooms quartered
1 aubergine roughly diced into small pieces
1 ½ cups dry green lentils rinsed
500ml water
2 veg stock pots
2 cans plum tomatoes
Large "glug" of (vegan) red wine
2 tablespoons balsamic vinegar
1 tablespoon of soy sauce
1 tablespoon of marmite
3 tablespoons of nutritional yeast
2 teaspoons of oregano
Salt and black pepper, to taste
Spaghetti of choice

Add the onions, carrots, celery and garlic into a pan with a splash of water in the bottom to start shallow frying and leave on a low heat to start to soften.

In the meantime add the aubergine to a smaller frying pan with a splash of water and fry on a medium heat to get really soft and almost sloppy then set aside.

Now your vegetables should be ready to start adding the lentils into the mix, water and stock pots. Leave this bubbling for 5 minutes on a medium high heat stirring frequently so they don't stick.

Now add your red wine, tinned tomatoes, soy, marmite, balsamic vinegar and 2 tablespoons of nutritional yeast, oregano and salt and pepper to taste.

Bring the sauce mix back to the boil, gently bubbling for 20 minutes, add your mushrooms and aubergine mix and cook for a further 10 minutes.

Remember to check the consistency of the sauce as the lentils may need a little bit more water depending on the thickness and how soft they are. If they still have a bite to them and the mix is getting quite thick add more water and one more stock pot if you feel it is necessary. I prefer my sauce to be slightly runnier.

Once you are happy with the sauce and the lentils are cooked through to your taste, serve on your choice of spaghetti and use the remaining nutritional yeast to sprinkle over as a plant based alternative to parmesan.

"I do hope you enjoy my recipes!" Natalie Sabih-Stone

Having enjoyed plenty of Natalie's recipes, I can personally vouch for how yummy they are!

#BlastOffTips

Laugh, smile and hug more

Hydrate

Exercise in the fresh air

Eat your leafy greens

12.
Rocket Fuel to Raise Your Vibration

So to recap......You create your own reality!

Similar to radio waves that are heard clearly but remain unseen, your vibrational frequency emanates from your cumulative thoughts, emotions and consciousness and is continually being broadcast out into the universe. This broadcast then attracts to you and mirrors similar experiences, people and opportunities, good or bad.

A high oscillating vibration attracts more high frequency, spiritually uplifting, or "positive" experiences in life. A low vibration attracts the opposite.

To determine your frequency, it's simple: pay close attention to your feelings. When you hold positive thoughts in your heart and mind, you feel happy, inspired and content; when you hold negative thoughts, you feel miserable, angry or sad. The better you feel, the higher your frequency will be; the worse, the lower.

As the creator of your life, the good news is you have the power to change your frequency and vibration at any moment. Even something as simple as laughing (laughter is the best medicine) or being creative can get the positive juices flowing.

Below are some timeless tips for raising your vibration, enhancing your manifesting success and experiencing more of the magnificent being that you are!

Practice Gratitude

Gratitude opens your heart and connects and aligns your energy to that which you love and is good in your life, attracting more of the same. It is a way to give (in its appreciation) and receive (through the opening created by that giving). The more you value and feel grateful for something, the more there will be to value. What you appreciate, appreciates!

In 2014, just before he passed away, I had the pleasure of meeting and listening to the internationally renowned Japanese scientist Dr. Masaru Emoto, author of The Hidden Messages in Water.

Dr. Emoto used high-speed photography to demonstrate how profoundly our thoughts, words and feelings impact molecules of water, the earth and our personal health. He found that water from clear springs and water that had been exposed to loving words like "thank you" showed brilliantly colourful, complex and multifaceted snowflake patterns. By contrast, polluted water and water exposed to negative thoughts formed incomplete, distorted and asymmetrical patterns with dull colours.

Imagine the effect saying thank you can have on our bodies, which are composed of over 70% water? To tap into the gratitude frequency, practice saying thank you to people in your life more regularly, and keep a daily gratitude journal listing everything you appreciate about yourself, your life and the world.

Drink Water

Water is an essential element for the survival of life. It is imperative to drink pure water in order to stay not just physically active but also to stay emotionally and spiritually stable. It is also considered that water is a form of the life force and energy.

The benefits of drinking pure water are well known. It can help you to maintain the clarity of the mind, it keeps you energized and it flushes out all the toxins from your body. All these result in increasing your vibration which ultimately leads to happy living.

In order to reap the most benefits of water, it's best to drink pure water. A great way to raise the vibration of the water is along the lines of what I mentioned earlier with the evidence from Dr. Emoto. Before you drink water next time, think of all the positive things and say "I love You Water" in your mind. This will infuse your water with positive qualities like love, peace and hope. Notice the difference when you do this next time.

Take Responsibility

Responsibility brings freedom and empowerment. The more you take responsibility for your life, the better able you are to change it. You create or allow all experience, whether you are conscious of it or not.

Become aware of the thoughts, feelings, beliefs and attitudes that are creating your world. Take responsibility for them and choose those that serve you and your world. Get excited about the future, own your power and get manifesting. You can move from victim to victor, from blame to gain, from fear or failure, to triumph and success!

Suspend Judgment

Judging others or yourself lowers your energy and separates you from love, truth and joy. It is a way of making yourself superior and above another by making them "less than" or "wrong", whilst projecting hidden guilt and self-attack on another.

The more you love and accept yourself, the less you judge others. We all make mistakes. Seek to forgive, understand and love both the one you are tempted to judge and any potential shadows within you that they are reflecting.

Smile

It is a scientific fact that the act of smiling releases "happy" chemicals into your brain that make you feel better which immediately raises your vibration. Smile and hold it for 10 seconds. Hold it and just see how you feel after. Notice your energy before and after you do this.

10 seconds. That's it. Feel your energy shift. Your brain doesn't know the difference between an outside event that makes you smile, makes you laugh, makes you feel joyful, and you just creating that experience.

So smile more often. Smile right now, as a matter of fact!

Forgive Yourself and Others

Forgiveness of self and others is the ultimate mind-body-soul detox. It liberates you from toxic emotions and sets you free from draining attachments. It can also dispel feelings of guilt, shame and undeserving that can otherwise block you from happiness and success.

It is an immensely powerful force for healing and transformation and a most gracious gift you can give yourself and another. (Chapter 9 Ho'oponopono!)

Show Kindness

Giving to someone else unconditionally i.e. without expecting anything in return shifts your thinking to "I have more than enough to give to others". Abundance is a high vibration.

In the same vein being kind (as opposed to being mean) puts you at a high vibration. As the saying goes, you get to keep what you give away.

The law of vibration states that any vibration which is sent out for good increases into higher frequencies as it moves through time and space until it returns to the sender, bringing with it the gifts of those higher frequencies.

In contrast any vibration sent out for selfish reasons such as greed or power will bring back vibrations with a lower frequency.

Perhaps you have heard the expression "give others what you desire the most". By giving others unconditionally that which you desire, you ultimately increase that which comes back to you.

Spend Time with Positive People.

It's been said that you become the sum of the five people you spend the most time with, so take a good look at your social circle and make sure it's elevating, not suppressing, your vibrational frequency.

Not sure if those around you are friends or frenemies? Take a look at how you feel and how you behave when you're with them. Are you your most authentic, empowered self, or do you put on a mask that disguises or demeans who you truly are?

After spending time with the friend or group in question, do you feel uplifted, empowered, and content? Or drained, angry, and depressed? Be honest, even if it means breaking with tradition and switching up your social circles. Your spiritual health depends upon it!

Watch Your Words

Every word you speak affects you at the quantum (energetic) level! The words you speak to others or yourself can actually be weakening your vibration and causing you to not feel good.

Your words guide your mind and body towards the experiences you want to have. For example, not saying anything negative for 24 hours will help you become more conscious about the things you say to yourself and to others. This is a wonderful challenge that you can do by yourself or with someone else. A lot of the times we don't even realize how many negative things we say.

Always keep the power of your words in mind. During your 24 hours start saying more kind things to yourself and others. Use your words to empower yourself, affirm exactly what you wish to experience, change the words you speak and you will raise your vibration.

Meditate

I've covered meditation already in Chapter 4 and in more detail (and how simply you can start) in Chapter 9, but please remember meditation has so many gifts, many of which are now being scientifically recognised and documented.

Meditation allows a calm and balanced perspective to be reached and negative states to dissipate and wash away as you centre and realign.

It also creates a gateway through which higher states of awareness can be reached, and the love and wisdom of your Higher Self more readily accessed. Meditation returns you to a place of clarity, truth and peace and allows your energy to clear and recharge.

Trust

Trust takes you towards happy desired outcomes in a magical, effortless way. Trust yourself and your power as a creator.

Trust the universe and the gifts it wishes to bestow open you. Trust the doors that are opening and those that are closing. Relinquish control and allow yourself to be carried along the river of trust, the universal flow, which take you to your goals with grace and ease.

Remember, the 2 passwords to the Fifth Dimensional portal (Chapter 6) Allow and surrender! And that takes trust!

Honour Your Emotions

Honour your emotions and listen to what they are telling you about what's going on inside. If they are negative or uncomfortable what thoughts or beliefs are they pointing to that may need changing or aligning?

Express and release your feelings rather than deny, repress, control or judge them. This doesn't mean wallowing in them or giving them undue attention if they do not serve you (i.e. nip that self-pity in the bud!), nor does it mean venting at someone inappropriately (writing a letter and burning it would be far "cleaner").

Honour your emotions by accepting them and allowing them to be experienced and released, be that by feeling them, writing them down, sharing them with a friend, or expressing them through creativity, for example.

Know You Are Loved

You are loved totally and unconditionally by the source of creation. There is nothing you need do to win that love and nothing you can do to lose it. Become aware of this truth and allow it in.

Open to receive this love. Doing so will enable you to experience more of your inherent value, increase your sense of worth and sense of deserving, heal pain of separation and loneliness, and experience more incredible love that is there for you in every moment.

Organise Your Environment.

Clear the clutter in your life! In fact every little bit of clutter is energy, and I cannot stress enough the importance of clearing the clutter at a very basic level in your home.

Clear the clutter and you energise your life! Do not live within a mass of paper, files, old boxes or piles of old magazines. Feng Shui is very powerful. You need to do it. Even if you spend ten minutes every day clearing a little bit, it'll make you feel so good and immediately raise your vibration.

If you are sad or depressed, clean out even one drawer. Our physical environment mirrors our emotional state; just as cleanliness is next to "godliness", a cluttered home is a sure sign of a cluttered mind.

Even chores as simple as taking out the rubbish, washing the dishes, vacuuming a room, or making your bed in the morning can have a measurable impact on your state of mind and provide an instant energy boost.

Contact a Feng Shui expert for guidance and help if necessary.

Move Your Body.

In addition to anti-aging, mood and metabolic benefits, even small amounts of physical exercise can raise your vibration.

Whether it's walking, running, swimming, spinning or practicing tai chi, qigong or yoga, physical exercise can help get you out of mental or emotional ruts and boost healthy endorphins.

It doesn't matter how much you sweat; the key is moving through and away from astral energies that could be weighing you down in your current environment.

Get out in Nature

If possible, exercise outside or somewhere in nature or by the sea. It truly does wonders reconnecting with nature and refilling our energetic batteries. Our bodies need natural light and natural air. Nature provides harmonic frequencies that are compatible with our personal frequencies.

Just noticing the trees, the natural sounds of birds singing, feeling your feet rooted in the grassy earth, breathing in fresh air and the pure positive source energy will help you transcend the concerns of what can perceived to be mundane human existence. This will reconnect you with your higher self which in turn raises your vibrational frequency.

Listen to Uplifting Music

Since music is a type of frequency, an audio frequency, you can easily raise your vibration by listening to music that feels good. It's an easy way to raise your vibration because it takes hardly any effort on your part to sit and enjoy a lovely tune.

Sound and vibration play a fundamental role in everything. Every object has a natural rate of vibration. In fact the human body is a symphony of sound; every organ, every muscle, every system, every bone, every cell no matter what size, are all in a state of vibration.

Listening to wonderful uplifting music can transform the most anxious hearts into compassionate loving ones full of positive energy. As you hear this music smile at your heart and see your heart as a flower, fresh, full of love and full of fragrance radiating out to the world.

Change your DNA

Did you know that your DNA has a vibrational frequency? Music recorded at 528 hz has been shown to resonate with the energy of love, peace and health. It is said to be the sound that resonates at the heart of creation. John Lennon used it when he recorded his song "Imagine".

Shower or Bath

Ever heard of people who get their best ideas in the shower? That's because cleansing helps wash away unseen energy patterns from the body's aura (including those picked up from others and accumulated throughout the day), making room for new creative thoughts and positive energies that are always seeking to guide us.

If you, like me, love a bath, just a twenty minute soak in some healing oils or Celtic sea salts can help detoxify your astral energy field, invigorate and soothe aching muscles. Where possible, use natural, organic soap free of toxins, artificial chemicals and fragrances (which weaken the aura). In a pinch, just washing your face and hands can help freshen your perspective.

For extra energy cleansing, try the Native American ritual of smudging with sage. Sage is a potent plant and burning it is a powerful ritual.

Burning sage (aka, "smudging" or "sage-ing") is a ritual used to "cleanse" a space or environment from negative energy, generate wisdom and clarity and promote healing. Intention is everything with this ritual, so before you light up, ask yourself what you're trying to purify, and/or heal from or release — inside you or in your space.

Use Crystals

Using large crystals in the home maintains high vibrational energy of your space and body.

Large crystals are the high vibration crystals because they hold the presence and energy of the earth. Earth energy reminds us to connect with the divine that created everything with the intention of love, compassion and abundance. Keeping high vibration crystals in each room will help foster a deeper spiritual life. Simply seeing a beautiful piece of the earth everyday will begin to transform your mindset.

Observe the night sky

On a clear night, gazing at the stars and other planets and observing the vastness of our limitless universe is hugely exhilarating and raises your vibration.

Unplug from the Matrix

Although computers, smart phones and ipads are great for staying connected in the information age, all electronic devices emit subtle, invisible electromagnetic fields (EMFs) that can negatively impact your energy field and drain spiritual life force.

To limit your exposure, use these devices for no more than two hours at a time before taking a break. At night before going to sleep, turn off all wi-fi equipment and even better unplug the router. If breaking with technology even for a few hours a day seems difficult, start small with a tech detox one hour a day, then just after work hours and eventually work yourself up to one tech-free day per week.

Go on a News Detox

Ever feel depressed, anxious or fearful after watching or reading the news? This is because most mainstream news outlets serve a primary purpose: earning profits. The quickest way to make a profit is by appealing to the lowest human common denominators of fear, greed and violence. As merchants of chaos, the mantra of "if it bleeds it leads" dictates what is, or is not newsworthy. As a result, a number of spiritual traditions recommend that seekers aspiring to higher states of consciousness refrain from reading and watching the news. Try it for a week and see how you feel. I personally rarely watch the news!

Clean Up Your Diet

A great way to increase your vibration is consuming foods that are filled with vital energy. Some foods vibrate at high frequencies and some lower. Most importantly pay attention to how eating certain foods make your body feel.

You've heard the saying you are what you eat. Remember every time you eat any kind of food you're absorbing its energy into your body. The quality of that energy has a direct impact on the quality of your health and vibration level. Energy is the core substance of everything in the universe, without energy there would be no life.

Understanding how energy frequency works is

important for your well-being. When your energy isn't vibrating correctly you are more vulnerable to diseases, negative thinking and depression. Plants are filled with vital energy from the sun which your body naturally understands. The more you consume high vibrating energy foods, the more positive, energized and vital you will feel, ultimately raising your vibration.

Serve Others

As the saying goes, you get to keep what you give away. Countless studies have shown that those who volunteer their time regularly towards worthy causes in service to others and the world are happier, healthier and more personally fulfilled.

The next time you are feeling overwhelmed or pressed for time to accomplish all of the tasks on your ever-growing to-do list, why not pay a visit to your local food bank, spiritual centre or homeless shelter and help out for an hour or two. Just the simple act of taking the focus off of your own problems and opening up to share with others will move you into greater alignment with the natural flow and grace of the universe.

Have Fun

Fun will attract success into your life like iron filings to a magnet. It is the antidote to stress, struggle, tediousness and seriousness. When you are having fun you are open and sharing of who you are and ride on the current of spontaneity and joy. What brings you fun, happiness and joy? Commit to more of it in all areas of your life!

Love, Love, Love!

Love yourself and others. There may be times this is easier than others, but make it your overriding intention. Love lies at the heart of all that you seek, and separation from it lies at the root of your troubles and pain.

Let love be a guiding light as you create a life filled with an abundance of love, happiness, joy, health and wealth.

We all love to love and be loved! It doesn't get better than that! It is the highest vibration there is. The more you love yourself and others, the happier, brighter and more fulfilling, purposeful and successful your life will become.

Wishing you peace, joy, love and light and of course

high vibrations on your amazing journey creating a life you love and beyond!

USEFUL SHEETS

For ease I've repeated the following sections by chapter at the back of the book so that you can cut or tear them out should you wish to!

Chapter 6 Rocket Fuel for Your Soul – Fifth Dimensional Living

Empowerment Prayer channelled from Archangel Gabriel

I AM myself

I accept myself

I value myself

I forgive myself

I bless myself

I express myself

I trust myself

I love myself

I empower myself

For all the times that I have given my power away to others or to fear, I call that power back to me NOW.

From this life or any other life, from this planet or any other planet, in this dimension or any other dimension ... hidden or seen ... I command my power back to me NOW.

Through every photon, atom, neutron and electron ... through every piece of my soul fragment; through my higher soul portal, I call back all my divine, empowerment NOW.

So just visualise now.....

Visualise waves of golden and white energy coming to you ...

breathe it in ...

allow the golden light of your empowerment to penetrate your skin ... cocoon you in light and open your solar plexus.

Feel your power returning to you ...

breathe it in ...

Feel your personal empowerment ignite with every breath you take ...

Feel your multi-dimensional DNA activate ...

and feel the acupuncture points on your body fill with photon packages of light, assisting your DNA to remember your unique spiritual powers and innate abilities

Bask in your divine empowerment light.

Radiate your light back to the Universe and throughout the planet.

Proclaim from this moment forward ... say out loud or to yourself....

Nothing can dim the light that I shine from within.

I have ignited my personal empowerment ...

and now just breathe it in ...

Feel your solar plexus open ... you have called back all the power that you have ever given away ...

And so it is ...

thank you, thank you, thank you

It is done, it is done, it is done

Chapter 8 Manifesting Abundance

Manifestation Oath

"I accept and receive unexpected good, unexpected money, unexpected love, unexpected kindness, unexpected generosity, unexpected offers, unexpected prosperity coming in unexpected ways from unexpected places in my life and the life of others.

I am constantly guided, and boldly empowered, to receive the lavish abundance of the Universe!

I accept the Principle that abundance and prosperity have already been given to me.

My acceptance makes it real and opens the space for manifestation to rush in!

I open wide the doors of my consciousness to receive and to give! It IS done now!"

Prosperity Prayer

Simply read it aloud with positive emotion every day for 40 days or longer if you feel you would like to.

"I am the source of all wealth. I am rich with creative ideas.

My mind abounds with new, original, inspired thoughts.

What I have to offer is unique and the world desires it.

My value is beyond reckoning. What the world needs and desires, I am ready to produce and give.

What the world needs and desires, I recognise and fulfil.

The bounty of my mind is without hindrance or limit.

Nothing can stand in the way of my inspired creativeness.

The over-flowing power of source energy overcomes every obstacle and pours out into the world, blessing and prospering everyone and everything through

271

me.

I radiate love,
I radiate blessings,
I radiate creativity,
I radiate prosperity,
I radiate loving service.
I radiate joy, love, freedom,
health, beauty, peace,
wisdom and power.

Humanity seeks me and rewards me. I am valued in the world.

I am appreciated. What I have to offer is greatly desired. What I have to offer brings a rich reward.

Through my vision the world is blessed.

Through my clear thinking and steadfast purpose, wonderful new values come into expression.

My vision is the vision for the greater good of all.

My faith is as the faith of the undefeatable.

My power to accomplish is unlimited.

I, in my uttermost source, am all wealth, all love, all health, all power, all productivity and all freedom.

I hereby declare my financial freedom NOW and henceforth forever!"

Chapter 11 Rocket Fuel For Your Body – Living Younger Longer

Recipes for Vitality

Good morning booster juice

Benefits - This is an overall powerhouse of a juice. All these amazing ingredients help to support and promote a healthy immune system, boost our body's natural detoxing abilities by removing toxins. This juice also can also help support healthier blood vessels and improve blood flow circulation.

You also get a wonderful hit of antioxidants from all those amazing colours which reduce inflammation and oxidative stress caused by diet, lifestyle and general everyday living. Not to mention the amazing cancer fighting properties that are in their too.

(2 days supply)
1 bag carrots

3 lemons
Large piece of ginger
2 turmeric roots
2 apples
2 whole raw beetroot
2 vine tomatoes
½ whole cucumber
2 celery sticks
¼ fresh chopped pineapple

Wash, prep and chop produce as necessary
Add produce to juicer one at a time
Stir well before drinking

Golden milk

Benefits Golden milk is an ancient Eastern tradition; it has been used in Ayurvedic medicine for centuries. The key ingredient is turmeric, a yellow spice popular in Asian cuisine which gives curry its yellow colour. The list of health benefits seems to be endless, it is mostly known for its anti-inflammatory effects which can help all types of joint pain such as arthritis due to its strong antioxidant properties.

This amazing drink can also support your immune system which helps to fight and protect your body from cancer, improve gut health and digestion. Not forgetting it has also been shown to support healthy blood sugar levels too.

(2 weeks supply)
100grams Ceylon cinnamon
100grams turmeric
1 teaspoon black pepper
2 tablespoons of coconut oil

In a pan, put the turmeric, cinnamon, the ground black pepper and half pint of water (for now). Bubble it all over a low heat stirring occasionally for about 15 minutes until it forms a sloppy paste, you may need to add more water to get that consistency.

Let the paste start to cool and then stir in the coconut oil.

Once cooled, pop into a jam jar or kilner jar, pop in the fridge and it will set. I use a large teaspoon every night in warm koko milk and the same every morning or mix in your superfood porridge for breakfast.

Superfood Porridge

Benefits A bowl of Porridge is such a great way to start your day! Not only does it provide a long lasting supply of energy, but oats have been proven to have powerful cholesterol lowering effects and can even help the body recover from certain cancers by removing excess hormones from our body.

The fibre present in porridge will leave you feeling fuller for longer and can help reduce the risks of naughty junk food cravings.

Incorporating blueberries and flaxseeds will help fire up the brain with healthy Omega 3 fats while supplying the body with a nice hit of antioxidants which can help fight free radical damage and prevent cancer.

By opting for a plant-based milk instead of dairy milk you instantly eliminate cholesterol and dramatically reduce the bad saturated fat from your diet, a far healthier way to go.

Choice of oats
Choice of plant based milk
Handful of blueberries
1 banana chopped
1 teaspoon golden paste (optional)
Sprinkle of flaxseed & linseed

Make your porridge as directed and then stir in the rest of the ingredients and enjoy.

Tasty Tomato Tostada

Benefits This Tostada will give you a nice hit of taste, colour and leave you feeling full and satisfied. It's also a great way to get some healthy fats from the avocado, antioxidants from the tomatoes and lemon juice in your diet. Not to mention the powerful cancer fighting properties from the red onion, garlic and coriander.

1 soft tortilla wrap
140g fresh sundried tomatoes diced
¼ red onion diced
1 avocado
Juice of ½ lemon
Small bunch of mint and coriander chopped
Salt and pepper
Vegan sour cream and Violife cheese (optional)
Fresh diced chilli
Handful of watercress

In a bowl mix the onion, tomatoes, mint and coriander. Mash the avocado until desired consistency; add the lemon juice, salt and pepper to taste and mix.

Pop the tortilla into a hot oven for 5 minutes to slightly warm. Once out, grate the Violife cheese onto it then sprinkle the tomato and onion mix all over leaving a space in the middle for the avocado.

I like to add my avocado mix to the middle and also sprinkle fresh chilli and then a few drops of the sour cream. You can either fold in half or eat open like a pizza with the watercress on the side.

Tabbouleh (gluten free)

Benefits This is a great way to get some healthy whole grains into your diet which play a key role in good health. Quinoa (which is technically a seed, however classed as a grain) was a staple in the Egyptian diet and is a well known source of good health.

It is loaded full of micro nutrients and is also a great choice of healthy carbohydrates, protein and fibre that will leave you feeling fuller and nourished for longer.

300g quinoa rinsed
2 vegetable stock pots mixed in 900ml boiling water
1 pack radishes thinly sliced
1 pack pomegranate seeds (between 200-300g depending on shop)
150g dried cranberries

3 sprigs of fresh mint chopped
Large handful of fresh parsley chopped
Large handful of fresh coriander chopped
Juice of 2 lemons

Add the quinoa to the bubbling stock water. Leave to bubble for about 30 seconds then lower the heat, add a tea towel fully across the top of your pot and replace the lid. Let it slowly cook, stirring occasionally. Around 12 to 15 minutes it should have absorbed the water and be fluffy and soft. Add the sliced radishes, pomegranate seeds, dried cranberries, chopped fresh mint, parsley and coriander and then squeeze 2 whole lemon juices over it and mix well.

Sweet Potato and Quinoa curry- medium spice

Benefits Not only is this dish full of flavour and colour but it will help fuel your body with the goodness that it needs. This dish also has an abundance of nutrients that can help support your immune system, lower cholesterol, balance your blood sugars and fire up your metabolism.

(Serves 4/6 as a side dish or 2 as a main)
300grams of quinoa – rinsed

600ml water
1 veg stock pot
1 red onion – diced
2 sweet potatoes – peeled and diced
250g frozen peas
2 teaspoons of garam masala
2 teaspoons of cayenne pepper
2 teaspoons of madras curry powder
2 teaspoons of cumin
2 tins chopped tomatoes
Salt and pepper to taste
1 teaspoon fresh garlic
Bunch fresh coriander
Sprig of mint
Alpro soya yoghurt (plain)
¼ whole cucumber grated

Peel and dice the sweet potato and lightly season with some extra garlic granules, cumin and cayenne and roast for 15 minutes or until soft.

In a pan fry the onions until slightly soft on a medium heat, add the quinoa, the veg stock pot, the water, all the spices, peas and the tinned tomatoes.

Gently bubble away on a low heat stirring frequently. You may need to add a touch more water depending on the cooking speed of the quinoa.

It takes about 20 minutes for the quinoa to cook with these extra ingredients to become light and fluffy but may need slightly longer. Mix in the cooked sweet potato, salt and pepper to season.

Sprinkle the coriander on top of the curry to taste. Mix the grated cucumber, yoghurt and chopped mint into a bowl for the cucumber raita and serve on the side.

Lentil Bolognese

Benefits This lentil bolognese is a great healthy alternative to the traditional minced meat version. By choosing a plant-based option you eliminate cholesterol and greatly reduced the bad saturated fat in your diet.

This heart healthy dish is loaded full of protein and a great source of carbohydrates that can help keep you leaner and full of energy, while helping to lower cholesterol and blood pressure.

(serves 4)
1 brown onion, diced
2 cloves of crushed garlic
2 large carrots, finely sliced

2 celery sticks, sliced
200g chestnut mushrooms quartered
1 aubergine roughly diced into small pieces
1 ½ cups dry green lentils rinsed
500ml water
2 veg stock pots
2 cans plum tomatoes
Large 'glug' of (vegan) red wine
2 tablespoons balsamic vinegar
1 tablespoon of soy sauce
1 tablespoon of marmite
3 tablespoons of nutritional yeast
2 teaspoons of oregano
Salt and black pepper, to taste
Spaghetti of choice

Add the onions, carrots, celery and garlic into a pan with a splash of water in the bottom to start shallow frying and leave on a low heat to start to soften.

In the meantime add the aubergine to a smaller frying pan with a splash of water and fry on a medium heat to get really soft and almost sloppy then set aside.

Now your vegetables should be ready to start adding the lentils into the mix, water and stock pots. Leave this bubbling for 5 minutes on a medium high heat stirring frequently so they don't stick.

Now add your red wine, tinned tomatoes, soy, marmite, balsamic vinegar and 2 tablespoons of nutritional yeast, oregano and salt and pepper to taste.

Bring the sauce mix back to the boil, gently bubbling for 20 minutes, add your mushrooms and aubergine mix and cook for a further 10 minutes.

Remember to check the consistency of the sauce as the lentils may need a little bit more water depending on the thickness and how soft they are. If they still have a bite to them and the mix is getting quite thick add more water and one more stock pot if you feel it is necessary. I prefer my sauce to be slightly runnier.

Once you are happy with the sauce and the lentils are cooked through to your taste, serve on your choice of spaghetti and use the remaining nutritional yeast to sprinkle over as a plant based alternative to parmesan.

ACKNOWLEDGEMENTS

In an intuitive moment with my great friend Claire I was guided to travel to Honfleur in northern France to write this book. Three separate trips later and *"The Power Within You Now"* was completed. Thank you beautiful Honfleur for your inspiration.

Huge love, gratitude and appreciation to my 3 children, Natalie, Rich and Nick for their wonderful contributions to this book and also to my great friend, Denise Sargent, for her beneficial contribution too.

Thank you to Victoria Jones for her proof reading, Michelle Catanach for the formatting and Mel Gwinnet for designing the cover.

I am also full of so much pride and gratitude for my amazing team within the Sue Stone Foundation. They have turned their expansive range of life challenges and obstacles into helping and supporting others from all walks of life.

I am also very inspired by the people around the world who have embraced these ideas, from whatever source, and applied them to their life. Thank you for tapping into positivity, possibility and potentiality and assisting in raising the vibration of our planet.

NOTES PAGE

NOTES PAGE

NOTES PAGE

NOTES PAGE

NOTES PAGE

NOTES PAGE

Notes Page

NOTES PAGE

NOTES PAGE

Notes Page